Perspectives in Lactation: Is Private Practice for Me?

Kathy Parkes, MSN-Ed, BSPsy,
RN, IBCLC, RLC, FILCA

Perspectives in Lactation: Is Private Practice for Me?

Praeclarus Press, LLC
2504 Sweetgum Lane
Amarillo, Texas 79124 USA
806-367-9950
www.PraeclarusPress.com

DISCLAIMER

The information contained in this publication is advisory only and is not intended to replace sound clinical judgment or individualized patient care. The author disclaims all warranties, whether expressed or implied, including any warranty as the quality, accuracy, safety, or suitability of this information for any particular purpose.

ISBN: 978-1-939807-50-2

Dedication/Acknowledgments

This book is dedicated to my husband, Bruce, who provided me with so many ideas about private practice and business, as well as this book. And to my daughters, Sarah and Jill, for the privilege of having them work for me at TLC, and for the fabulous suggestions through the years. I love "all y'all"!

I want to publically thank the mothers and babies I had the privilege to work with over those 15 years of TLC operations. Friendships were formed, and I learned a tremendous amount of information about the breastfeeding relationship from them. I value those experiences more than those moms and babies will ever know. And I met my mission statement, "To change the world, one mother and baby at a time."

Gratefulness and heartfelt thanks go out to all the lactation professionals I have worked with over the years. The sharing, feedback, and shoulders mean more to me than you realize. I am who I am today partially because of you.

Table of Contents

Introduction

I've learned that people will forget what you said, people will forget what you did, but people will never forget how you made them feel.

–Maya Angelou

When I began my first private practice in 1993 as an International Board Certified Lactation Consultant and Registered Nurse, the climate was ripe for this type of service. In a city of 1.5 million people, nearly a dozen hospitals delivered tens of thousands of babies each year. There was only one other private lactation practice in town that provided only office visits. It was the best of all worlds to begin a practice. The Lactation Connection (TLC) Inc. began as a separate room in my house for consultations and breast pump rentals. Within a year, I was driving over one hundred miles each day, five to six days a week, to provide home consults and pump deliveries. TLC had over 100 breast pumps for rent to those in need. By year five of practice, TLC moved out of my house and opened a small office in a business park and was seeing four to five consults each day, renting and selling products, and had a contract with the city's Women's, Infants, and Children's (WIC) program to provide monthly inservicing to staff and peer counselors. Within another five years, TLC tripled the office space, was providing a wide variety of weekly classes, and bringing in a second IBCLC to provide multiple consults at the same time. TLC was thriving and was known throughout the area as a high-quality, patient-friendly, and research-based service provider.

At the same time, though, private practice lactation consultants (PPLCs) around the country began to notice a climate change for practice. Hospitals were hiring more and more IBCLCs, beginning their own lactation centers, and capturing their resident populations for consults, pump rentals, and product sales prior to discharge. Many PPLCs were reducing services, cutting back on rental and sale products, or even closing their doors. TLC noted the same climate change locally. The number of private pay patients declined, pump rentals went from 200 per month to less than 50, especially when pump companies developed high-quality single-user breast pumps and made them available in big box stores. Increasing numbers of locations were renting breast pumps, including durable medical equipment companies, drug stores, and even baby item stores. Of course, no knowledge of the product or teaching on use went with those rentals, but the city was over-run with rental depots.

In response, TLC went back to offering home visits, while trying to maintain a large office space. I reduced products and was returning rental pumps to the companies by the dozens. Within months, the outside office was closed. After 15 years in practice, TLC closed its doors, as did the other PPLC in the city. Every hospital in San Antonio that delivered babies had their own lactation center with products, rentals, and lactation consultants, some of whom were IBCLCs with years of practice. The climate had changed completely.

Several years ago, I began my second private practice, with a focus on local, state, national, and international speaking, teaching, assisting businesses with Mother Friendly practices, and online consults. Breastfeeding Perspectives™ is slowly growing, and I am enjoying this new focus of private practice. It is due to my own experiences, both positive and negative, that I came to write this book.

In preparation for this book, I designed a survey and sent it to approximately 50 lactation consultants in private practice. Those who returned the survey ranged from new practitioners to those who have been in practice for 30 years. Thanks go out to these lactation consultants who shared so freely. Their answers to the survey questions may help you avoid some of the lessons they learned the hard way. The survey questions and their responses appear throughout the book in boxes entitled "Experienced LCs Share." The final question is shared in Chapter Fourteen.

Hopefully, you will find information in this book to assist you in building your own private practice and enjoying the ownership of a small business. I would love to have feedback on your experience; contact me at Kathy@breastfeedingperspectives.com.

Chapter One. Am I Ready for Private Practice–Education, Experience, Credentials?

Never doubt that a small group of thoughtfully committed citizens can change the world. Indeed, it's the only thing that ever has.

~Margaret Mead

Many lactation consultants enter private practice with excitement and the anticipation of building a large clientele and having the freedom to practice without the restrictions frequently placed on them in a healthcare setting. The expectation of bringing in large sums of money to cover a salary, conference costs, and resources, such as new books and continuing education materials, looms large in their minds. They may have no business plan or accounting background, and may not have prepared for working long days, nights, and weekends. The work of advertising, getting the word out, and networking has not been planned or put down on paper. And the potential for being on-call 24/7 is far from their minds.

Building a private practice as a lactation consultant is one of the hardest things you will ever do. It will drain you physically, emotionally, psychologically, and possibly monetarily. It will take time away from your family, more than you expect. Is it worth it? Absolutely! But you'll want to do your homework and plan exhaustively, something this book will attempt to assist you in completing. So let's start at the very beginning.

What is a lactation consultant?

At this time, there is no registered copyright on the term "lactation consultant." Anyone can call themselves by this term. However, there are two American Nurses Credentialing Center (ANCC)-approved classifications for certification of lactation consultants. The ANCC's Nursing Skills Competency Program recognizes the importance of high quality continuing nursing education (CNE) and skills-based competency programs (http://www.nursecredentialing.org/Mission-Statement). The first, most-well-known, and highest practice standard is the **International Board Certified Lactation Consultant®** (IBCLC®), which has been an integral part of the healthcare field for over 25 years. The International Board of Lactation Consultant Examiners® (IBCLE®) is the independently accredited international certifying organization conferring the IBCLC credential. As of the 2013 IBCLC exam, there are over 26,500 IBCLCs in 96 countries around the globe. The International Lactation

Consultant Association® (ILCA®) is the professional association for IBCLCs and other healthcare professionals caring for the breastfeeding family and has a current membership of more than 6000. ILCA advocates the promotion, protection, and support of breastfeeding for all mothers and infants, and supports the IBCLC in doing so. The IBCLC is the only internationally recognized credential in the field of lactation, and assures families, employers, insurers, and policy makers of competent, evidence-based lactation care and services.

Lactation consultants may find work in a wide variety of locations, including hospitals, clinics, physicians' offices, WIC clinics, neonatal intensive care units, human milk banks, and private practice. The IBCLC credential can be a stand-alone credential or an add-on to another currently held credential, such as a Registered Nurse. At this time, about 80% of the IBCLCs in the United States are also RNs. This is not the case in many other countries, where physicians and midwives hold an IBCLC as an add-on credential.

According to the *Position Paper on the Role and Impact of the IBCLC*, there are nine roles served by the IBCLC. These roles include: **advocate** for breastfeeding women, infants, children, families, and communities; **clinical expert** in the management of breastfeeding and human lactation; **collaborator** with mothers, infants, children, families, communities, healthcare teams, and policy makers; **educator** to provide evidence-based information and anticipatory guidance on breastfeeding and human lactation; **facilitator** for meeting breastfeeding goals, as well as program and policy development; **investigator** to support, direct, and participate in research and evidence-based practice on lactation; **policy consultant** for institutional and legislative initiatives that influence breastfeeding; **professional** in a multi-disciplinary role for breastfeeding and allied health care; and **promoter** to support and protect breastfeeding (ILCA, 2011).

The background experiences of IBCLCs vary, but each candidate must have education in specified health-science subjects (biology, human anatomy and physiology, infant and child growth and development, nutrition, psychology, counseling, research, sociology, basic life support, medical documentation and terminology, occupational safety and security, ethics, and universal precautions and infection control), education in human lactation and breastfeeding, and clinical practice in providing care to breastfeeding families. Candidates should have a broad range of clinical experience in providing lactation and breastfeeding care that spans the spectrum from pre-conception through weaning, and encompasses an extensive variety of clinical skills. All IBLCE examination candidates are required to report lactation-specific clinical practice hours that were obtained within the five years immediately prior to applying for the examination. The number of hours that are required will depend upon the pathway being followed, from 300 to 1000 hours. Following the completion of these requirements, candidates must sit a rigorous, independent, criterion-referenced exam to be awarded the IBCLC certification. Recertification must take place every five years in order to maintain the IBCLC credential. Recertification by exam is always an option for candidates, but is mandatory every ten years. Recertification by continuing education can be completed at the five-year interval, with 75 CERPs necessary. Fifty of the 75 CERPs must be lactation specific, five must be in professional ethics, and the remaining 20 are to be relevant to the lactation consultant profession. Recertification ensures a commitment to excellence in practice, provision of current research-based care, and protection for the consumer of lactation services.

Standards of practice "describe what is considered 'best practice' by the profession to ensure a consistent quality of performance that protects public health, safety and welfare" (ILCA, 2013). These standards of practice "promote consistency by encouraging a common systematic approach; are sufficiently specific in content to guide daily practice; provide a recommended framework for the development of policies and protocols, educational programs, and quality improvement efforts; and are intended for use in diverse practice settings and cultural contexts."

IBCLCs, as allied healthcare providers, are expected to adhere to the following practice documents (ILCA, 2013):

- ILCA Standards of Practice for International Board Certified Lactation Consultants (voluntary)

- IBLCE Code of Professional Conduct for IBCLCs (mandatory)

- IBLCE Scope of Practice for International Board Certified Lactation Consultant Certificants (mandatory)

- IBLCE Clinical Competencies for the Practice of International Board Certified Lactation Consultants (mandatory)

- The International Code of Marketing of Breast-Milk Substitutes (mandatory)

- All subsequent, relevant World Health Assembly Resolutions, as it applies to health workers, whether legislated (mandatory) or not (voluntary)

These professional standards and guidelines make the IBCLC the gold standard in the lactation profession.

However, currently there are various credentials that bring confusion to the consumer, healthcare provider, and legislator. These certifications include CBE (certified breastfeeding educator), CBS (certified breastfeeding specialist), CLS (certified lactation specialist), LS (lactation specialist), LLLL (accredited Leader with La Leche League International), BC (breastfeeding counselor with Breastfeeding USA), NMC (accredited leader with Nursing Mothers' Council), PC (WIC peer counselor), CLE (certified lactation educator), LEC (lactation educator certified through CAPPA), and CLEC (certified lactation educator counselor).

The second ANCC credential for lactation consultants is the **Certified Lactation Counselor®** (CLC®), offered through the Healthy Children Project and recognized by ANCC as a Nursing Skills Competency Program. CLCs have successfully completed a 45-hour training and passed a criterion-referenced examination. No college courses or clinical lactation practice hours are required to fulfill the exam requirements. Demonstration of competencies and skills required to provide evidence-based education and counseling for pregnant, lactating, and breastfeeding women must also be shown. More than 13,000 CLCs have been certified by the Healthy Children Project in the United States. CLCs can be found providing basic lactation care in hospitals, community clinics, physician offices, and private practice. To practice, they agree to comply with the Scope of Practice and the Code of Ethics for CLCs from The Academy of Lactation Policy and Practice (TALPP). Certification expires three years after passing the exam and can be renewed with 18 hours of continuing education. No prior nursing or medical degree or training is required to receive the CLC certification, although many recipients use it as an add-on credential. According to the Healthy Children Project website, many "are L & D nurses, NICU nurses, mother baby nurses, public health nurses, LPNs, doctors, nutritionists, speech language pathologists, occupational therapists, doulas, peer counselors, midwives, perinatal outreach workers, and volunteer breastfeeding counselors" (www.healthychildren.cc). The CLC certification is a stepping-stone to the IBCLC credential.

The Healthy Children Project also offers certificates for Advanced Nurse Lactation Consultant and for Advanced Lactation Consultant. People receiving these certificates must recertify every three years and complete 25 hours of continuing education.

In 2014, the United States Lactation Consultant Association (USLCA) published "Who's Who In Lactation? An Inventory of Breastfeeding Support: From Confusion to Clarity." The full document is available at www.uslca.org. Here is the table provided within the document, outlining various breastfeeding titles, the training time necessary, and the skills needed to be accredited, certified, or verified.

Table 1.1. USLCA Who's Who in Lactation

TITLE	TRAINING TIME	SKILLS
International Board Certified Lactation Consultant (IBCLC)	Approximately 5 years of preparation	90 hours lactation specific education 8 college level health professional courses (24 academic credits) 6 health related continuing education courses 300-1000 clinical practice hours Pass a criterion-reference exam The International Board Certified Lactation Consultant possesses the necessary skills, knowledge, and attitudes to provide quality breastfeeding assistance to babies and mothers. The IBCLC specializes in the clinical management of breastfeeding which includes: preventive healthcare, patient education, nutrition counseling, and therapeutic treatment. http://iblce.org/certify/eligibility-criteria/
Certified Lactation Counselor (CLC)	45 hours	This comprehensive, evidence-based, breastfeeding management course includes practical skills, theoretical foundations and competency verification. Certification is accredited by the American National Standards Institute. www.healthychildren.cc/clc.htm
Certified Lactation Specialist/ Breastfeeding Specialist	45 hours	Designed for the aspiring lactation consultant or nurses, physicians, midwives, dieticians, breastfeeding assistants or others desirous of improving their knowledge base and skills in working with the breastfeeding dyad. This certification is a stepping-stone to the IBCLC credential. www.lactationeducationconsultants.com/course_clsc.shtml
Lactation Educator Counselor	45 hours	This university based program trains participants to be Lactation Educator Counselors. Lactation Educator Counselors are typically entry level practitioners and deal primarily with the normal process of lactation. This course is the required prerequisite to the Lactation Consultant course. http://breastfeeding-education.com/home/clec-2/

Breastfeeding Counselor	10-14 months, Provide 30 hours of support	2-3 day workshop, self-evaluation, one written paper & case studies, read and review 5 books, submit one survey on breastfeeding support available in their community, open book online tests (multiple choice) to cover physiology & anatomy. http://childbirthinternational.com/information/pack/htm
Breastfeeding Counselor	Approximately 9 months of self-study	Breastfeeding Counselors (BCs) are accredited representatives of Breastfeeding USA who participate in mission-related activities in their communities, online, and with the national organization. A mother who has breastfed her baby for at least one year and fulfills the other personal experience requirements can become a BC by successfully completing the application and education program. Breastfeeding Counselors understand the significant role that mother-to-mother support plays in women's overall success and satisfaction with breastfeeding. Accordingly, their primary function is to offer evidence-based breastfeeding information and support to women through in-person meetings, by phone, or online as representatives of Breastfeeding USA. Other examples of mission-based services include providing administrative support to volunteers, participating in advocacy activities, and translating materials into other languages. www.breastfeedingusa.org
Lactation Educator Certification	120 hours online training, includes 50 hours health science 75 hours self-directed study/mentorship	Qualified to teach, support, and educate the public on breastfeeding and related issues and policies. Workbook activities, required reading materials, attend breastfeeding meetings, research paper, submit a class presentation, work for clients in their community. www.birtharts.com/lactation-educator-certification.htm
Community Breastfeeding Educator	20 hours	Does not issue Lactation Consultant status. For community workers in maternal child health, focuses on providing services to pregnant women to encourage the initiation and continuation of breastfeeding. www.healthychildren.cc/maternalinfant.htm/
Baby Friendly Curriculum	Approximately 20 hours	Used by facilities to strengthen the knowledge and skills of their staff towards successful implementation of the Ten Steps to Successful Breastfeeding. www.babyfriendlyusa.org/get-started

WIC Peer Counselor	30-50 hours, Varies by state, some states have quarterly training	Peer counselors are mothers who have personal experience with breastfeeding and are trained to provide basic breastfeeding information and support to other mothers with whom they share various characteristics, such as language, race/ethnicity, and socioeconomic status. In WIC, peer counselors are recruited and hired from WIC's target population of low-income women and undergo training to provide mother-to-mother support in group settings and one-to-one counseling through telephone calls or visits in the home, clinic, or hospital. Refers mothers with challenging questions and concerns to an IBCLC. www.nal.usda.gov/wicworks/Learning_Center/support_peer.html
Certified Lactation Educator	20 hours total, some have 8 hours clinical	Qualified to teach, support, and educate the public on breastfeeding and related issues. Complete course training, attend support group meetings, observe consultation or videos, review research studies and other requirements, including a test. www.cappa.net/get-certified.php?lactation-educator
La Leche League Peer Counselor (volunteer)	18-20 hours	Have successfully breastfed their infants for 6 months. Program developed to provide support systems within targeted communities that will provide ongoing access to breastfeeding information and support. www.llli.org/llleaderweb/lv/lvaugsep99p92.html
La Leche League Leader (volunteer)	Approximately 1 year of self-study training	An experienced breastfeeding mother, familiar with research and current findings dealing with breastfeeding, who offers practical information and encouragement to nursing mothers through monthly meetings and one-to-one help. www.lalecheleague.org/lad/talll/faq.html.#howlong

---

Experienced LCs Share

What degrees and work experiences did you bring into your practice?

The private practice lactation consultants answering the survey comprised a wide variety of backgrounds prior to opening a lactation practice. Many are registered nurses with experience in labor and delivery, postpartum, normal newborn, and neonatal intensive care units.

There are those who had Associate, Bachelor, or Masters Degrees in fields outside of lactation and nursing, ranging from communications to biology to theatre to education.

One IBCLC who holds a Masters in Library Science said, "My paid work experiences were all in various types of libraries, where I learned that the first question someone asks is not really the question they want answered. The first question is a 'test' question. If you answer that question in a manner to their liking, they will then ask the question they 'really' want answered. It works that way at the library reference desk and with breastfeeding mothers!" Definitely a sage piece of advice for all lactation consultants.

Also represented were midwives, doulas, massage therapists, WIC Peer Counselor trainers, WIC Breastfeeding Counselors, and childbirth instructors. Interestingly enough, 80% of the current U.S.-based IBCLCs are RNs first, according to ILCA.

Where can I get reliable lactation education?

The Lactation Education Accreditation and Approval Review Committee (LEAARC) provides a voluntary approval process to lactation education programs who have existed for more than one year, have been offered more than one time, offer a minimum of 45 contact hours, cover areas of the IBLCE Exam Blueprint, and have a faculty who have been IBCLC certified for more than five years (www.leaarc.org). As of this writing, 25 courses have been awarded the LEAARC approval, providing educational readiness for the IBCLC exam. These include:

- Arizona State University–57 hour Southwest Clinical Lactation Education Program (www. https://nursingandhealth. asu.edu/lactation/southwest-clinical-lactation-education-program?destination=node/3797)

- Birthingway College of Midwifery–107 hour Lactational Consultant Program (www.birthingway.edu/breastfeeding-counselor-and-lactation-consultant-programs.htm)

- Breastfeeding Outlook–90 hour Comprehensive Lactation Course: Mastering the Blueprint (www.breastfeedingoutlook.com/index.php?pageID=113)

- Breastfeeding Support Consultants–200 hour distance learning Lactation Consultant Course (www.bsccenter.org)

- Bright Future Lactation Resource Centre Ltd.–45 hour Lactation Management/Exam Preparation Course (www. BFLRC.com)

- California State University, Northridge–45 hour Lactation Education course (www.csun.edu)

- The Centre for Breastfeeding Education–102 hour Lactation Medicine Programme (www.institute.nbci.ca)

- County of Riverside Department of Public Health–105 hour Grow Our Own Lactation Consultant Program (www. lovingsupport.org/growourown)

- Danish Committee for Health Education–90 hour Interdisciplinary Breastfeeding Course (www.sundkom.dk)

- Deborah Robertson, IBCLC–120 hour Breastfeeding Specialist Course (www.breastfeedingspecialist.com)

- Diffusion Allaitement–90 hour Human Lactation Program (www.allaitement.net).

- Douglas College–77 hour Breastfeeding Course for Health Care Providers (www.douglas.bc.ca)

- Health e-Learning-IIHL–120 hour BreastEd Online Lactation Studies Program (www.health-e-learning.com)

- Healthy Children Project, Inc.–45 hour Lactation Counselor Certificate Training (www.healthychildren.cc)

- The International Institute of Human Lactation, Inc.–119 hour Lactation Education Program (aussiecan@videotron.ca)

- Lactation Education Consultants–46 hour Certified Lactation Specialist Course (www.lactationeducationconsultants.com)

- Lactation Education Resources–45 hour Lactation Consultant Training Program (www.lactationtraining.com)

- Lactation Education Resources–90 hour enriched Lactation Consultant Training Program (www.lactationtraining.com)

- Mohawk College of Applied Arts and Technology–132 hour distance learning breastfeeding program (www.mohawkcollege. ca)

- Northwest Area Health Education Center–69 hour North Carolina Lactation Educator Training Program (www.northwestahec.org)

- Portland Community College CLIMB Center for Advancement–45 hour Lactation Management in the 21st Century Program (www. pcc.edu/climb/health)

- ProMAMA Center Association—90 hour Education in Lactation Program (www.consultant-lactatie.ro)

- University of California San Diego, Extension—128 hour Certificate for Lactation Consultant Program (www.breastfeeding-education.com)

- Wichita State University School of Nursing—45 hour distance learning program (http://webs.wichita.edu/?u=CHP_NURS&p=/HumanLactationOnline/index/)

How can I keep up-to-date in the industry?

Mothers nowadays are being discharged with infants who are gestationally younger, weigh less, have complicated sucking and feeding difficulties, and present with many more issues to lactation consultants than 10 or 15 years ago. Late preterm infants go home at four or five pounds, at a gestational age that doesn't always allow for effective milk transfer. Many more mothers are conceiving infants through methods that involve hormones and may not have effective milk productions. Private practice lactation consultants are seeing more women with breast augmentation; not necessarily a problem until you delve further to find out they had no breast tissue to begin with. There are more unusual situations, such as surrogacy, transgendered, same-sex marriages where both mothers want to breastfeed, mother-to-mother milk sharing, visually or hearing impaired mothers, and the list goes on and on. As a private practice lactation consultant, you will be seeing what are commonly referred to in professional lactation circles as "train wrecks," those mothers and infants who have worked with lesser-practiced lactation providers and been told there is no hope for them. They have complicated problems and need long-term solutions and support.

It is vital as a lactation consultant in private practice to keep your skills and research-based knowledge top-notch. You should plan to attend conferences regularly, join professional organizations to receive the peer-reviewed journals, buy the latest issues of the most necessary reference books, be online with other lactation professionals, and participate in local, state, national, and/or international lactation organizations, taskforces, coalitions, etc. Your practice and your reputation depend on this.

Appendices A and B provide a listing of state, national, and international breastfeeding organizations. Appendices C, D, and E provide listings of professional organizations and resources, research sites, and email lists and blogs.

Experienced LCs Share

How long had you been an IBCLC before going into private practice?

After passing the IBLCE exam and becoming an IBCLC, over half of the respondents hung out a shingle as a private practice lactation consultant immediately. Most had prior experience as a La Leche League Leader or other mother-to-mother breastfeeding support leader, a hospital nurse, or other healthcare provider.

Those that did not do so immediately upon passing the exam opened their private practice within six months to ten years.

Private Practice Self-Check

Do you have the education needed that makes you competent and eligible to open a private practice? If not, what education do you need?

Do you have the credentials needed that make you competent and eligible to open a private practice? If not, what credentials do you need?

Do you have the experience needed that makes you well practiced enough to open a private practice? If not, what experience do you need?

Chapter Two. Do I Have an Entrepreneurial Personality?

Don't aim for success if you want it; just do what you love and believe in, and it will come naturally.

–David Frost

Bank of America recently released their Small Business Owner Report (2013) for the spring of 2013. Did you know that only 21% of small business owners (SBO) are spending more time with a spouse, family, or friends; only 35% of SBOs are exercising more frequently; only 29% are eating healthier; only 49% of SBOs get between seven and eight hours of sleep every night; 72% of SBOs work more than 40 hours each week; and the time a small business could survive a disruption before needing outside financial help is only five months? The top factors affecting the success of small businesses over the next 12 months are a combination of recovery of consumer spending (76%), consumer confidence (75%), current tax environment (67%), strength of the U.S. dollar (59%), commodities pricing (59%), effectiveness of government leaders (58%), healthcare costs/benefits (56%), and availability of credit (52%). All of these factors are beyond your control.

According to the blog, "How Long Does It Take To Become Profitable?" (2011) at www.entrepreneuideadads.com, the average for start-up small companies to see a profit is three to five years. Only one-half of new businesses survive at least five years, and only one-third survive to the ten-year point (SBA, 2012).

Are you scared yet? If not...

Do you fit the entrepreneurial typecast? How do you know?

Books on the business of owning a small business revealed several factors in personalities that increase the potential of success as a business owner. Can you multitask as the owner, CEO, accountant, marketing specialist, webmaster, writer of policies and procedures, and trainer of employees?

Do you crave thrills, excitement, and speed? Are you a highly creative problem-solver? Are you intuitive, ambitious, and industrious? Are you high-energy, driven, a risk-taker, a leader, intelligent, a positive thinker, and a goal-setter? Do you have a burning desire to be successful? These are the most commonly mentioned personality traits of a successful entrepreneur.

Do you tend to procrastinate? Are you easily distracted? Are you irritable? Do you have addiction problems? Are you listless or depressed? Do you have a fear of success? These are personality pitfalls that might cause you to fail as a business owner.

The Internet has multiple sites with free entrepreneurial personality tests. If you can answer them honestly, you can receive a great deal of information about yourself in the profiles presented. *The DaVinci Method* and other books by Garrett LoPorto provide follow-up for the initial personality tests provided free online (www.davincimethod.com).

Heart, Smarts, Guts, and Luck (wwww.hsgl.com) is one of the websites with a personality test. The authors Anthony Tjan, Richard Harrington, and Tsun-Yan Hsieh took the results of research on hundreds of successful entrepreneurs and business-builders and narrowed the information down to four main decision-making styles–heart, smarts, guts, and luck–that determine success in business. They developed the Entrepreneurial Aptitude Test to help people figure out which of these traits dominates their personality and decision-making style. Understanding your dominant traits will help you determine if you have what it takes for long-term success in the business world. They have also written a book on the subject (Tjan, Harring, & Hsieh, 2012).

There are dozens of other personality tests available; just use your search engine to find "entrepreneur personality tests" and you can spend hours taking the tests!

Business owner Gayle Santana (2014) described the ways to be successful concluding that the number one way is to be committed. In her experience, regardless of the business, the journey is always the same. "It's a long road of self-examination and improvement, skill examination, and education. It's making judgment calls about people, things, and situations." She says you need to trust your gut, keep the faith, and stick it out in tough times. You don't quit just because money is low. She says commitment to the journey is the key to business success (Santana, 2014).

Do you have the commitment to make your business work? If so, you can overcome any obstacles in your personality and be a successful business owner. It may take hard work, it may take a partner who has the traits you are missing, but you can make it work if you are committed!

Private Practice Self-Check

Do you have the personality to be a business owner?

What traits do you have that will make you a successful business owner?

What traits do you have that might hinder you as a business owner?

How can you offset any traits that might hinder you?

Do you have the commitment to create and run a successful business?

Chapter Three. Is the Business Environment Right for My Business?

I don't measure a man's success by how high he climbs but how high he bounces when he hits bottom.

~George S. Patton

OK, I've got the education, experience, and credentials, and the entrepreneurial personality. Now what?

Business Environment

The next step should be to perform some research on the business environment in your area. What are the birth rates in your area? How many hospitals provide birthing units, and do they have their own lactation centers? Do they provide post-discharge follow-up with their patients? What is the availability of other private practice lactation consultants in the area you plan to cover? Is there sufficient opportunity for growth and expansion of your practice in this area?

The U.S. Census Bureau completes a nationwide accounting every two years. Two exceptional websites provide statistics from the census: www.quickfacts.census.gov and www.censusviewer.com. On these sites, you can find interactive maps, demographics, and facts about towns, cities, counties, and states. Population is broken down by age, gender, race, income, families with children, those on food stamps or welfare, education, occupation, religion, and zip code. These sites also include information on small businesses. In addition, many towns and cities maintain online statistics for births, population makeup, income, and other facts and figures.

The biannual Maternity Practices in Infant Nutrition and Care (mPINC) survey is administered by the Centers for Disease Control (CDC) to every hospital and birthing center with registered maternity beds in the United States and Territories. The latest published results are for 2011; the 2013 survey is currently being completed as of this writing. The CDC survey covers labor and delivery care, postpartum feeding of breastfed infants, breastfeeding assistance, postpartum contact between mother and infant, facility discharge care, staff training, and structural and organizational aspects of care delivery. These results can be accessed at www.cdc.gov/breastfeeding/data/mpink/index.htm and are compiled by national and state results. Each hospital and birthing center receives their own scores for that location, which are not published for the public. Although you may not have the mPINC details for hospitals and birthing centers in the area you wish to cover as a private practitioner, the mPINC can provide ideas regarding services provided in your area, as well as the services which could be provided in your practice.

What are your chances of running a successful private practice in your area? A thorough understanding of your target market and the current economic conditions are keys to the growth and success of your private practice. The Small Business Administration (www.sba.gov) is an excellent source for providing information during your research. The SBA website contains general business data, statistics on business type from small to large firms, economic indicators, detailed labor statistics, employment projections, wage data, financial statistics, and information about women in the labor force. Spending time on this aspect of research is critical. You may have the most experience of any lactation professional in your area, but if the economic atmosphere is poor, your private practice could be an effort in wasted time and money with little to no income.

Once you have a potential location in mind, consider joining any local breastfeeding committees, task forces, or coalitions that are available to you. At these meetings, you can meet others in the lactation support field, find out if there is a need for the services you want to provide, and network with those who could potentially refer clients to your practice. Lactation consultants often participate in these groups. You can discuss with them how to best support the services they already provide and what types of services they think are needed. Remember, competition is not a threat; it enables you to think outside the box and provide services not available at other locations. A listing of breastfeeding coalitions is included in Appendix B.

Speaking of Money...

How much money will you need to start your private practice? Where will it come from? Do you have collateral for a bank small business loan?

SCORE (www.score.org) is a large group of volunteer mentors. On this site you can get free business tools, templates, tips, and confidential business counseling if you are starting a small business or growing your established business. Free and inexpensive business workshops are offered in over 340 local chapters, and webinars are available online 24/7. The start-up forms contain information on protecting your business ideas, how to write a strong business plan, a complete financial and planning gallery, how to set up a home-based business, and what tax breaks you may claim. They also provide information about being adequately insured in your business and available financing locations.

To establish your initial start-up expenses, you will need to include advertising, inventory, cash on hand, decorating, fixtures and equipment necessary (use actual bid figures), liability and professional insurance, rental payments, licenses and permits, professional fees (renewing your nursing license, your IBCLC fees for recertification, ILCA membership fees), CPA, attorney, etc., telephone, Internet, cleaning, accounting, etc., signs, and supplies (from pens and paper to cleaning supplies). Be sure to include a contingency fund for coverage of the unexpected. You will need a working capital fund, as you cannot open your practice with an empty bank account. Make sure this fund is adequate to cover those first months in practice when more funds go out than come into the business. The recommendation for working capital is at least three to six months of complete business costs, including your salary.

Experienced LCs Share

Regarding the start-up monies used for your practice, was this your own investment, a business loan, or something else? Approximately how much was your start-up cost?

No business loans were used to begin any of the practices in this survey. All IB-CLCs used either their own funds or a loan from a family member. Start-up costs ranged from $1000 to $7500 to open the practice doors and begin seeing clients.

Monies used for startup can come from a variety of sources, the first being your own pocket. The more money you can invest in your practice up front, the less you will need to finance, with the accompanying interest and financing costs to cover in your monthly payments. Arrange a sit-down meeting with the small business professionals at multiple banks in your area. Find out if they can provide all the services you need. Compare those services with each other and choose the most appropriate institution for your needs. Questions might include topics such as interest rates on loans, interest rates on savings accounts and money market accounts, and credit card services for your business, both for you to make purchases from your suppliers and for you to accept payments from clients.

Check online for small business loans for women-owned businesses from federal and state governments. Often, they provide funds at a lower interest rate than local banks or credit unions. The Small Business Administration (SBA) can provide your practice with the certification of a "woman-owned business" and can provide multiple loan options. A Women-Owned Small Business (WOSB) Federal Contract Program is offered to help level the playing field for contracting with the federal government, which can prove to be extremely helpful for a one-person private practice in lactation.

Will I have a Return on Investment?

A return on investment (ROI) is a way to measure the profit earned from each investment, be it time, energy, skills, or money. The Business Dictionary (2014) defines ROI as "a measure of profitability that indicates whether or not a company is using its resources in an efficient manner." Generally, you will want to measure the amount of gross profit minus the investment, and divide that by the investment. For example, if you are measuring marketing, it would look like this:

Gross Profit – Marketing Dollars Invested
Marketing Dollars Invested

You could also measure your social ROI, which includes the value of human resources, using qualitative, quantitative, and financial information. For assistance with premade formulas, search the Internet for SROI.

The return on investment can be used within your practice to measure performance on pricing policies, inventory investment, or employee wages versus earnings. The ultimate objective is to remain in the black when figuring the ROI.

Morningstar.com lists rates of return according to industry (2014). Depending on the type of industry lactation consultants would be categorized within, the rates of return vary. As of November 28, 2014, the ROI for Education & Training Services was 1.63 for one year, three year was -0.21, and five year was -4.70. Within the Health Information Services, one year ROI was 1.08, three year was 12.98, and five year was 15.05. If you consider your practice personal services, ROI for one year was 9.76, three year was 13.34, and five year was 13.35. If your practice carries products for sale, you might fit the specialty retail category and expect a one year ROI of 3.43, three year of 17.63, and five year of 18.94. To calculate your own return on investment, research the industry you feel your particular practice falls into. The Internet is replete with data to use in this calculation.

Private Practice Self-Check

Can your area support a private practice lactation business?

How will you fund your business?

If you need a loan, are banks in your area willing to make loans for small businesses?

If no, what other resources are available to fund your business?

Will you be able to see a return on your investment?

Chapter Four. The Legal Requirements of Being in Business

Some people dream of success while others wake up and work hard at it.
~ Winston Churchill

It has been said by experienced private practice lactation consultants that unless you have a degree in business, you are never fully prepared for the number of business decisions you will have to make regarding your practice on a daily basis. From filing the appropriate "doing business as" paperwork, deciding if you want to be a sole proprietorship or a partnership, to filling out all the tax paperwork and keeping accounting records. Designing reports to file with healthcare professionals, deciding how long, legally, you must keep all records, figuring out the legalities of HIPAA, figuring out the Affordable Care Act and its effect on your practice, marketing your practice; the list seems never ending and very confusing.

Experienced LCs Share

What do you wish you had known prior to going into private practice?

Many of the IBCLCs reported not feeling prepared for the business side, such as accounting, paperwork, billing, reimbursements, insurance, and knowledge of state or county-wide requirements for private practice.

Not being aware of the pros and cons of partnership and other business entities was mentioned as a negative for making that particular choice.

Business Structure

Your first order of business is to establish what your practice structure will look like. Choices abound and entire books are available on this topic. Here are some basics:

Sole Proprietorship: This is the easiest and most popular business structure, usually involving only one individual who owns and operates the entire business. As owner, you are financially and legally responsible for the practice, including debts and obligations related to your business. As owner of a sole proprietorship, you have unlimited liability, meaning that should a creditor raise a claim or a client file a lawsuit against your practice, you are placing all your assets at risk, both business and personal. Securing capital for starting the business may be more difficult as a sole proprietor. You will report all business income and losses on your personal income tax return, using Schedule C Profit or Loss from Business, along with your personal 1040. Self-employment tax should be filed quarterly in four equal amounts on the 15th of April, June, September, and January. If you hire an employee, social security and Medicare taxes must be withheld from their paycheck and filed with the IRS (Form 941 Employer's Quarterly Federal Tax Return, Form 944 Employer's Annual Federal Tax Return, W-2 Wage and Tax Statement, W-3 Transmittal of Wage and Tax Statements). An annual tax payment for Federal unemployment tax (FUTA) is filed on Form 940. All forms can be found online at www.irs.gov, along with instructions for each. A direct link is also provided to individual state tax requirements.

Advantages	Disadvantages
• Low start-up costs	• Unlimited liability
• Greatest freedom from city/state/federal regulations	• Difficulty in finding capital funding
• Owner has full control in decision-making	• No one to take on the practice if owner is unavailable
• Profits flow to owner	• No name protection
• Use of business revenues as desired	
• Tax advantages	
• Dissolution relatively uncomplicated	

Source: Small Business BC (www.smallbusinessbc.ca.)

Partnership: Like the sole proprietorship, a general partnership has unlimited liability. Two or more people are involved in this business venture, with clearly defined responsibilities outlined in a partnership agreement. Each owner shares in the management of the business, is personally liable for all debts and obligations of the entire practice, and assumes the consequences of the other partner(s) actions. In a limited partnership, one or more partners provide only capital, without control or legal liability for the company. Taxes must be filed by the partnership on Form 1065 Return of Partnership Income. Employment taxes are filed using Form 941 Employer's Quarterly Federal Tax Return and Form 940 Employer's Annual Federal Unemployment (FUTA) Tax Return. In addition, each partner files Schedule F Supplemental Income and Loss and Schedule SF Self-Employment Tax with their individual income tax Form 1040. Partners are not employees and do not need Form W-2, but copies of Schedule K-1 should be furnished to each partner.

Advantages	Disadvantages
• Shared entrepreneurial experience • Pooled resources • Practice profits flow directly to owners • Lower start-up costs • Easy to form • More sources of investment funding • Limited regulation	• Formation costs more expensive than sole proprietorship due to need for legal and accounting services • Personal liability for actions of all owners • Divided authority among owners • Potential for conflict between partners • More complicated to dissolve • No name protection

Source: Small Business BC (www.smallbusinessbc.ca.)

Corporation: A corporation is a legal entity that is separate and distinct from its owners/ members/shareholders. Legal distinction is made between the company and its owner(s), keeping the owner from being liable if a lawsuit is filed. Forming a corporation is more complex and expensive than a sole proprietorship or partnership. Debt acquired within a corporation is not considered a personal debt of the owner and personal assets are not at risk. Profits in a corporation can be retained without the owner having to pay taxes on them. Investment capital is more available to corporations. However, owners of the company must pay a double tax on the business earnings through personal income taxes at federal and state levels and shareholders' earnings (dividends), which are taxed on their personal tax returns. A special type of corporation, the S Corporation, provides business owners with limited liability for the company, but they do not pay income taxes. Rather, the corporation's income and losses are passed along to its' shareholders. Income taxes are filed on Form 1120 Corporation Income Tax Return, and estimated taxes on Form 1120-W Estimated Tax for Corporations. If the corporation has employees, employment taxes for social security, Medicare, and federal unemployment (FUTA) must be filed on Form 941 Employer's Quarterly Federal Tax Return and Form 940 Employer's Annual Federal Unemployment (FUTA) Tax Return.

Advantages	Disadvantages
• Limited liability to owners	• Highly regulated at federal and state levels
• Separate taxes from owners	
• Company exists in perpetuity	• Most expensive business type to form
• Ownership is transferable	• Extensive record keeping necessary
• Investment capital more obtainable	• Possible for shareholders to be held legally responsible
• Separate legal entity	• Extensive reporting to shareholders
• Easy to transfer business	• Complex formation
• Name protection	• Required Articles of Incorporation which is matter of public record
	• Possible ongoing incorporation fees

Source: Small Business BC (www.smallbusinessbc.ca.)

Limited Liability Corporation (LLC): An LLC is a hybrid of a sole proprietorship and a corporation, providing limited liability for the owners and taxation only once on the business. However, this business structure is defined by individual state statutes and many contain different regulations. Check your state regulations regarding formation of an LLC. Owners in an LLC are called members, and the types of members are usually not limited. Individuals, corporations, other LLCs, and even foreign entities may be members. The maximum number of members is not regulated, and many states permit a single-member LLC to form with only one owner. Taxation by the Internal Revenue Service will vary depending on the elections made by the LLC and the number of members. An LLC with two members is classified as a partnership for federal income tax purposes unless it files Form 8832 Entity Classification Election to be treated as a corporation. An LLC with only one member is treated as an entity disregarded as separate. The income from an LLC still gets claimed on the owner's personal income tax filing for income tax purposes, but the LLC is treated as a separate entity for purposes of employment tax and certain excise taxes. Once again, Form 8832 can be filed to treat this entity as a corporation.

Advantages	Disadvantages
• Limited liability	• Difficulty with investment capital
• Flexible tax structure	• State regulations vary
• Less red-tape than corporation formation	
• Flexible management of company	

Source: Small Business BC (www.smallbusinessbc.ca.)

Experienced LCs Share

What do you wish you had known prior to going into private practice?

Many discussed the importance of developing a logo and a business name, and branding with colors and text prior to beginning consultations.

Naming Your Practice, Filing Your DBA, Obtaining an EIN

When choosing a business name (the legal wording is fictitious name) for your private practice, choose a name that appeals to you and to the type of customers you are trying to attract. Consider names with an emotional connection that will appeal to potential clients. Stay away from long, complicated, or confusing names, and from "cute puns" that only you understand. The word "Inc." cannot be used after your name unless your company is actually incorporated, and the word "Enterprises" commonly demonstrates amateur status. Be creative and unique. Pick a name that has not been claimed by others, online or offline. Check to see if a website address or URL is available for your potential business name. Think about how your name will appear as part of a logo and marketing materials. Search the U.S. Patent and Trademark Office using their free search tool to see if a similar name or variations on it is already trademarked. If the name is already trademarked, choose another name. Trademark infringement can carry a high cost for your new business.

What is a trademark? It is the right to use a specific name, word, phrase, symbol, logo, design, combination of letters or numbers, sound, or color scheme to identity your intellectual property, making it stand out from other products. Your unique name is a common law usage and can be used with the ™ symbol; however, protection for common law marks is limited. Trademark laws provide protection from competitors stealing your identity or using a name or symbol so similar that it could be confused with yours in the minds of clients and customers. It also protects customers from deceptive practices by others. One way to protect your business name is to register a trademark. To register a trademark, file with the U.S. Patent and Trademark Office; pricing for paper filings begins at $375 and for electronic filings at $325. Upon approval of the registration, you can begin to use the ® symbol behind your business name. No common or generic terms (for example, breastfeeding) can be trademarked. Trademarks must be renewed every ten years.

Claiming your social media name should take place early in the naming process. Although it may be too early to know what social media sites you will be using for your practice, it is a good idea to go ahead and secure the name. You may want to use it later. More on your Internet presence appears in Chapter Ten.

Once you have decided on a business name and structure for your practice, you may need to file a DBA or "Doing Business As." As a sole proprietorship, the DBA is required if your business has a different name than your own name. This is the simplest and least expensive way to use your business name. You need a DBA to open a bank account and receive payments in your business name. For corporations and LLCs, the paperwork formation for the entity provides registration of your business name, and a separate DBA is not necessary. However, filing a DBA allows you to operate multiple businesses without having to form a separate LLC or corporation for each business. Contact your town/city/county clerk's office for details on whether your practice needs to file a DBA since regulations vary by county and state. The Small Business Administration (www.sba.gov) provides a chart that details filings for DBA from state to state. Many private practitioners have found that working with a legal filing system or a lawyer assures that they are following all applicable county and state requirements to prevent operating outside the law.

The Employer Identification Number (EIN), also known as a Tax Identification Number (TIN), is used by the IRS to identify a business entity required to file various business tax returns. The number is issued only once to your business and does not have an expiration date. Sole proprietorships may not need an EIN, since the owner's social security number is used on tax filings. For other business structures, though, an EIN is necessary to pay employees or file business tax returns. Many financial institutions will not open a business account without the EIN number. Unlike a social security number, the EIN is not sensitive information. Many businesses freely distribute their EIN in marketing materials, advertisements, and websites.

Applying for an Employer Identification Number can be done quickly and free of cost at the IRS website's online application process. After answering a series of questions, your EIN confirmation notice can be downloaded, saved, and printed immediately. Be sure to check with your individual state for regulations regarding a state EIN or charter.

Experienced LCs Share

What legal paperwork did you have to file for your city, county, state, or country?

Federal, state, county, and city paperwork was filed by the majority of these private-practice LCs. National Provider Numbers, business licenses, Employer Identification Numbers, property tax assessment, Doing Business As for business name filings, state tax identification numbers for taxes to be paid on retail sales, and state small business licenses were all included.

Several LCs mentioned obtaining professional malpractice and liability insurance prior to beginning practice, which is highly recommended.

For lactation consultants holding licenses in other professions, annual renewals through fees and continuing education have to be made for each profession.

Two IBCLCs also filed the extensive paperwork to be recognized as in-network providers for insurance companies.

The extensive time and monetary fees for each of these items should be taken into consideration for those wishing to go into private practice.

Small, Minority, and Women-Owned Business Certifications

Federal, state, and city governments offer assistance to minority and women-owned small businesses, which can be advantageous in landing business contracts. Most public corporations, as well as governmental purchasing agencies, have programs allotting a certain percentage of business to women and minority-owned small businesses. The major time investment necessary to become certified may affect whether or not you will want to gain this additional business advantage. The requirements for submitting an application for certification are stringent and must be met completely. Collecting the extensive paperwork necessary to apply may seem overwhelming, unless you can be VERY organized from the moment you begin to run your business.

To be eligible for the Women-Owned Small Business (WOSB) program, the business must be at least 51% owned, controlled, and managed by one or more women, and the women must be U.S. citizens. The business must be "small" in accordance with the Small Business Administration's (SBA) size standards for that industry. Four organizations have been approved by the SBA to act as Third-Party Certifiers for the WOSB Program. These are the El Paso Hispanic Chamber of Commerce, the National Women Business Owners Corporation, the U.S. Women's Chamber of Commerce, and the Women's Business Enterprise National Council (WBENC). Owners may elect to certify through one of these four agencies or go to the SBA website to file electronically. In addition, many cities and states offer local certification to women business owners. For example, if you plan to do business with the local hospital in your city, the scope of your business practice would not require a national certification. If you desire to land a federal contract with a governmental agency, you will want to contact individual agencies to obtain their certification requirements. Rules may vary from state to state, and many agencies require that WOSB owners obtain certification through their program because they maintain their own regulations.

Minority-Owned Small Businesses (MOSB) can receive SBA 8(a) certification through the National Minority Supplier Development Council (NMSDC). To comply with the SBA's 8(a) Business Development Program, 17 states and 25 cities, as well as an impressive list of corporations (IBM, Microsoft, Marriott, etc.), accept NMSDC certification for programs designed to help minorities win public-sector contracts. U.S. for-profit businesses of any size can apply if they are owned, operated, and controlled by minority group members who are U.S. citizens. Fifty-one percent of the business stock must be owned by a minority member. For purposes of the NMSDC's program, a minority group member is one who is at least 25% Asian-Indian, Asian-Pacific, Black, Hispanic, or Native American heritage. NMSDC has designated 37 regional councils to provide a standardized application for certification.

The Minority-Owned Business Program exists in most cities and states, often referred to as Minority Business Enterprise (MBE) programs. One excellent example is Austin, Texas. Their website (www.austintexas.gov) provides resources for small and minority businesses, current contract opportunities, MOSM and WOSM reports, vendor connections, and three types of certification for small and minority-owned businesses. These are Minority- and Women-Owned Business Enterprise Certification, Disadvantaged Business Enterprise Certification, and Small Business Enterprise Certification. Free monthly workshops are offered on becoming certified and how to do business with the City of Austin.

Laws Affecting How You Practice

The Health Insurance Portability and Accountability Act (HIPAA) of 1996

HIPAA is a U.S. federal law that (1) limits the ability of a new employer plan to exclude coverage for preexisting conditions; (2) provides additional opportunities to enroll in a group health plan if you lose other coverage or experience certain life events; (3) prohibits discrimination against employees and their dependent family members based on any health factors they may have, including prior medical conditions, previous claims experience, and genetic information; and (4) guarantees that certain individuals will have access to and can renew individual health insurance policies. Included in the 115 page bill are the Administrative Simplification provisions that require the Department of Health and Human Services (HHS) to adopt national standards for electronic healthcare transactions and code sets, unique health identifiers, and security. At the time of passage of this bill, Congress recognized that advances in electronic technology could erode the privacy of health information. In December 2000, HHS published a final Privacy Rule, later modified in August 2002. This Rule sets national standards for the protection of individually identifiable health information by health plans, healthcare clearinghouses, and healthcare providers who conduct healthcare transactions electronically. In February 2003, a final Security Rule was published by HHS, setting national standards for protection of confidentiality, integrity, and availability of electronic-protected health information. This privacy rule, "The Standards for Privacy of Individually Identifiable Health Information," addresses the use and disclosure of individuals' health information, as well as setting standards for individuals' privacy rights to understand and control how their health information is used.

As a lactation consultant, you do not fall under the categories of covered entities listed in the HIPAA documentation, health plans, or healthcare clearinghouses. However, you may fall under the healthcare provider as a covered entity if you electronically transmit health information in connection with certain transactions. These include claims, benefit eligibility inquiries, referral authorization requests, or other transactions for which HHS has established standards under the HIPAA Transactions Rule. This covers healthcare providers whether they electronically transmit these transactions directly or use a billing service or other third party to do so on their behalf. Healthcare providers include all "providers of services," "providers of medical or health services," and any other person or organization that furnishes, bills, or is paid for healthcare.

Protected Health Information (PHI)

HIPAA's Privacy Rule protects all "individually identifiable health information" (protected health information or PHI) held or transmitted by a covered entity in any form or media, whether electronic, paper, or oral. PHI is information, including demographics, that relates to the individual's past, present, or future physical or mental health or condition, the provision of healthcare to the individual, or the past, present, or future payment for the provision of healthcare to the individual.

HHS Office for Civil Rights (OCR) is responsible for administering and enforcing these standards and may conduct compliance investigations and reviews. Covered entities that fail to comply voluntarily with the standards may be subject to civil monetary penalties. These penalties range from $100 to $50,000 or more per violation, with an annual cap of $1.5 million. In addition, certain violations of the Privacy Rule may be subject to criminal prosecution with monetary fines and imprisonment.

As a covered entity, the privacy standards for PHI include information located in verbal or written communication; computer files or paper patient files; information shared with other healthcare providers, payers, consultants, attorneys, or other third parties; or information transmitted or maintained in any other form of media.

Your practice must inform clients of their rights related to PHI. To address this requirement, there are certain documents and forms that need to be provided to each client, including a notice of privacy practices (Notice), and authorization. The Notice informs clients how their PHI may be used by the practice and explains their rights. Reviewing this Notice provides the client with the opportunity to talk about any privacy issues or concerns she may have. The practice must be able to show that this Notice has been provided to the client. The Authorization form for the use and disclosure of specific PHI should be signed by the client. Authorizations should be obtained for uses and disclosures that are not related to treatment, payment, and healthcare operations. Samples of notices of privacy practices can be found in English and Spanish at http://www.hhs.gov/ocr/privacy/hipaa/modelnotices.html

To help make sure the Notice is provided as required, HIPAA identifies situations that would require a Notice. These include:

- The Notice must be available at locations where healthcare services are provided.

- The Notice must be provided at the first visit or encounter. If the initial services are provided at the request of a patient who is not physically present (for example, an online consult), an electronic copy of the Notice must be provided.

- A copy of the Notice must be posted in the facility in areas where clients will likely see and read it.

- If the practice maintains a web site, a copy of the Notice must be posted and readily available.

- Additional copies of the Notice must be provided to the client upon request.

The American Recovery and Reinvestment Act (ARRA) expands each client's privacy rights under HIPAA. Under these rules, clients may choose to not file a claim for payment with their group health plan if the individual pays out-of-pocket for a healthcare service. They may request and receive information in electronic format if the information is maintained as an electronic health record at a reasonable cost for complying with the request. And they may receive an accounting of PHI electronic disclosures for treatment, payment, and healthcare operations during the previous three years. Therefore, you should have written policies and procedures in place regarding client rights.

How can lactation consultants comply with the Privacy Rule? One way is encryption, the act of changing electronic information into an unreadable state using algorithms (mathematical rules) or ciphers. Originally used for passing highly classified government and military information electronically, the general public is now entering personal, sensitive information over the Internet. The secure server on various websites automatically encrypts text when consumers click into the site. Sensitive data should be encrypted, and as private practitioners, LCs are encountering this on a daily basis. What is considered sensitive data? Full name, Social Security number, credit/debit card numbers, billing and shipping addresses, bank account and bank account log-in information, financial and salary information, driver's license number, date of birth, health and patient information, and student information.

According to www.csoonline.com, David Kilgalion says, "No security solution will protect sensitive data completely." Increasingly intelligent hackers are everywhere, and all companies should work under the principle that their data will be compromised at some point. Encryption can soften the blow by making the data unreadable without an encryption key or set of characters or instructions that algorithms use to encrypt/decrypt information. The cost of encryption is far less than the financial and HIPAA repercussions of a data breach.

The Health Information Technology for Economic and Clinical Health (HITECH) Act, part of the American Recovery and Reinvestment Act of 2009, made several important changes to the HIPAA Security Rule. One change is the requirement for HIPAA-covered entities to provide notification in the event of a breach of "unsecured protected health information (PHI)." If the computer database, laptop, tablet, PDA, or smart phone of the LC in private practice is compromised (stolen, hacked, etc.), you need to notify the affected clients and the Department of Health and Human Services (HHS).

The HIPAA Security Rule is a three-tier framework of Safeguards, Standards, and Implementation Specifications. Within the Technical Safeguards, both the Access Control Standard (data at rest) and Transmission Security Standard (data in motion) have an Implementation Specification for Encryption. Neither of them is "required," but both are listed as "Addressable." The HHS states, "In meeting standards that contain addressable implementation specifications, a covered entity will do one of the following: (1) Implement the addressable implementation specifications; (2) Implement one or more alternative security measures to accomplish the same purpose; or (3) Not implement either an addressable implementation specification or an alternative." So encryption is not required; however, the HHS states, "a covered entity must implement an addressable implementation specification if it is reasonable and appropriate to do so, and must implement an equivalent alternative if …it is unreasonable and inappropriate, and there is a reasonable and appropriate alternative…The decisions that a covered entity makes regarding addressable specifications must be documented in writing. The written documentation should include the factors considered, as well as the results of the risk assessment on which the decision was based" (www.hhs.gov/ocr/privacy/hipaa/faq/securityrule/2020.hmml).

For a lactation practice, what does all this mean? Basically, you are required to encrypt PHI in motion and at rest whenever it is reasonable and appropriate to do so.

Manual encryption involves selecting appropriate files to run through the encryption program. According to the SANS Institute (2003), one common mistake business owners make with manual encryption programs is that they will encrypt their data, but leave the un-encrypted version accessible. Some programs provide the option to automatically delete the original document after it has been successfully encrypted. Apple's policy regarding the storage of data on iCloud states that the information is encrypted when being sent and while contained on the server (http://support.apple.com/kb/HT4865).

File encryption programs range in price from free to well over $200.00. Lifehacker.com recently listed their five favorite encryption tools as being GNU Privacy Guard (for Mac/Linux, free); Disk Utility (for Mac, free); TrueCrypt (Mac/Linus, free); 7-zip (free); and AxCrypt (free). A quick Google search for encryption software showed dozens of possible software programs, as well as encrypted thumb drives, external encryptors, and more.

The Affordable Care Act ("ObamaCare")

Health insurance reform legislation, "The Affordable Care Act," was passed by the U.S. Congress and signed into law by President Obama on March 23, 2010. Under this act, women's preventative healthcare services generally must be covered by health plans with no cost sharing. Regarding lactation, the ACA states, "Breastfeeding support, supplies and counseling: Comprehensive lactation support and counseling by a trained provider during pregnancy and/or in the postpartum period and costs for renting breastfeeding equipment will be covered in conjunction with each birth" (http://www.hhs.gov/healthcare/facts/factsheets/2011/08/womensprevention08012011a.html).

This is a broad statement, providing payment by the insurance company for anyone providing any support to a breastfeeding mother. "Regulations prevent insurance companies from deciding who should receive this payment; it is not an arbitrary process. In order to be recognized as a 'trained' provider, the usual standard is a medical license. In order to participate in an insurance company's network of providers, you must go through a rigorous credentialing process, by regulation, standard, and law. In order to pass the credentialing process, you must have an identified credential" (Susan Madden, COO, National Breastfeeding Center; www.NBFCenter.com).

Private Practice Self-Check

What business structure have you chosen for your business?

___ sole proprietorship ___ partnership ___ corporation ___ limited liability corporation

What name (DBA) have you chosen for your business?

What web address, Facebook page name, Twitter name, and/or other social media names have you reserved for your business?

What is your Employer Identification Number (EIN)?

How will you comply with HIPAA requirements?

How will you inform your clients of their rights related to PHI?

How will you meet the American Recovery and Reinvestment Act privacy requirements?

Will you apply to insurance companies to be recognized as a trained provider under the Affordable Care Act?

Chapter Five. What Type of Office Should I Have?

I wish I may, I wish I might, have the wish I wish tonight.

~ 19th century American nursery rhyme

Opportunities for private practice lactation consultants abound. You can establish a practice from your home, provide consultations solely in the client's home, or have a brick-and-mortar office outside of your home. Contracts have been written by private practice LCs with hospitals, the offices of local Women, Infants, and Children (WIC) programs, and public health clinics. Home healthcare practices will sometimes contract with or hire a lactation consultant. More and more frequently, physician practices are hiring part-time or full-time lactation consultants for their clientele. And with new technology developing every day, private practice LCs are also offering online consults for mothers around the world. In Indiana, Walgreens Drug Stores have contracted with IBCLCs to provide consultations, pump rentals, bra sales, and other services for breastfeeding mothers in their facilities.

Home-Based Offices

Home-based small businesses are the rule rather than the exception. Money is a primary reason for starting out in a home-based office, as many home-based entrepreneurs start with less than $5,000 and no savings for their businesses. Adapted from an article on home-based businesses (McCall, 2000), here are some suggestions to consider when starting a home office for your practice:

Is your home accommodating to clients? Do you have dogs, cats, or birds that can provoke allergies, make noise, or scare little ones? Make sure you can close out the home noises to your office.

Will your office space allow for expansion as you add clients and/or equipment? Think about the space needed for printers, scanners, fax machine, more file drawers, a baby changing station, scale for infant weights, comfortable seating for various sized mothers, and more.

Can you dedicate your office space to business only? You will need to keep the business phone off limits to others, especially children, be able close the door to the office at the end of the day, dedicate the computer and other equipment to business use only, and allow no intrusions into the office space during consult time.

Can you keep your business and personal life separate? There are often many distractions in the home and in the business that may not allow you to separate one from the other. If you do decide to have a home business, the business phone line should always be answered professionally, with your business name and your personal name. You will need to obtain a P.O. box where you receive all business mail. Don't use your home address for your business cards, forms, or other documentation. Without a storefront, your image is important. Professional business cards and forms can help provide a professional impression.

While working from a home-based office may provide many advantages (no commute, lower start-up fees, increased tax write-offs, more flexibility in work hours, and more family time), there are distinct disadvantages. Space may be at a premium, personal and family life may be continually disrupted, and there is a lack of social contacts and networking. Stress levels are increased due to the need to balance family and business life since many lactation consultants have a hard time walking out of the office and leaving "work at work."

There are zoning laws, homeowners' association restrictions, and building regulations that need to be researched prior to opening your home office. To assist in deciding whether you need to seek governmental permission on home offices, ask yourself these questions: (1) Will my home no longer be used mainly as a private residence? (2) Will my business result in a marked increase in local traffic? (3) Will my business involve any activities considered unusual for a residential area? (4) Will my business disturb my neighbors at unreasonable hours? If you answer yes to any of these questions, you need to seek permission from one or more governmental agencies.

Zoning laws are applicable to home-based businesses. There are restrictions on physical changes to the appearance of your home, including exterior physical changes for the purposes of conducting business; prohibition of outside business activities, storage, or displays; and restriction or prohibition of signage. Traffic restrictions are included in most zoning laws, limiting the number of visitors to a home-based business, restricting the number of employees, and restricting business parking. Most zoning codes also restrict or prohibit nuisance impacts, such as noise, odors, or glare, as well as prohibiting the storage of hazardous materials.

To prevent neighborhood complaints to the zoning board, you will want to be proactive in researching your residential zoning, mercantile, vendor, fire, and other ordinances that could affect a private practice. Call or visit your local municipal building and request a copy of the laws that apply to home occupations. Or check the municipal website, as many cities are now placing their entire code book online for researching by interested parties. Start at the lowest level, such as your lease if you currently rent your home, and with the covenants and restrictions for your homeowners association. These supersede any county laws within an incorporated city.

Hearings for special exceptions or variances can be requested, depending on the type of business you want to operate. You must be able to prove "no impact" to receive the variance or exception, with no increased traffic, no outside visitors, and no outside evidence that there is a business on the premises. Be aware that applying for a municipal variance can be costly ($5000 to $50,000), time-consuming, and frustrating. An additional drawback to receiving a variance is the commercial site regulations your home then falls under. This means it can be inspected at any time of the day or night without notice or a warrant for fire code violations and compliance with OSHA, Americans with Disabilities Act, and other commercial business regulations. These inspections can be costly, requiring fire doors, ramps, ADA compliant toilets, fire prevention sprinkler systems, and more to be added to your residence.

The Internal Revenue Service (IRS, 2013) provides guidelines for deductions to be claimed for a home-based office. This 24 page document can be downloaded free from the IRS website. Generally, you cannot deduct items related to your home, such as mortgage interest, real estate taxes, utilities, maintenance, rent, depreciation, or property insurance as business expenses. However, you may be able to deduct expenses related to the business use of part of your home if you meet specific requirements. Even then, the deductible amount of these types of expenses may be limited. To qualify for deductions, you must use part of your home exclusively and regularly as your principal place of business where you meet or deal with patients, clients, or customers in the normal course of your trade or business. In the case of a separate structure not attached to your home, you may be able to qualify for deductions if you use it in connection with your trade or business on a regular basis for certain storage use or for rental use. Your Certified Public Accountant can help you to claim these deductions appropriately if you meet the criteria set by the IRS.

Home Visits

Private practice lactation consultants frequently offer consultations in the comfort of the mother's home. Issues like insurance coverage for general and professional liability, forms to use, and vaccination status still apply when providing home visits. There are several additional concepts to keep in mind.

Being solo, autonomous, and on your own for the majority of the day occasionally proves challenging for LCs doing only home visits. It is refreshing or taxing, depending on your personality and methods of "filling your own emotional tank." Taking advantage of this alone time to dictate notes and impressions into a mobile device can be helpful. Parking in a beautiful spot and entering consult notes into your laptop or iPad can be energizing. You will want to carry snacks, lunch, and/or water to take care of your own needs. For many, the temptation for fast food at the drive-through window is strong. This becomes unhealthy and expensive if done on a regular basis, and as a business owner, your goal is to make money.

Your personal safety is of utmost concern when providing services in the mother's home. Consults may be provided in neighborhoods where conditions might not be ideal. Someone should always know where you are going, how long you plan to be there, and have a way to contact you. You may occasionally walk into a home where domestic violence is present. Carrying a mobile phone, iPad, or other device with a GPS can help to call for assistance or locate you in times of trouble. Do not leave expensive equipment in plain site within your vehicle, as thieves may take advantage of your two-hour consult.

What should you take with you to a home consult? Minimum recommendations include a high-quality scale (Medela Baby Weigh, Tanita); feeding devices (LactAid, SNS, 25cc syringe and #5 French feeding tubes, periodontal curved-tip syringes, nipple shields, spoons or feeding cups); teaching materials (books, photos, videos, and websites available on laptop or iPad, written handouts, fabric breast); professional items (name or identification badge; lab coat or scrub jacket; non-latex gloves and finger cots; clean towels and washcloths; hand sanitizer; sanitizer for equipment cleaning between consults; penlight; forms; laptop or iPad; business cards; credit card scanner, such as Square; cell phone; paper; and pens); and resource availability list (pump rentals if you do not provide them; nursing bras; La Leche League or Nursing Mothers Council meetings; breastfeeding and birthing classes; doulas; healthcare providers for frenotomy, physical therapy, craniosacral work, massage, chiropractic work, and breast surgery; and LC specialists). If you take professional photos of unusual lactation situations, be sure to have a good camera and a release form for client consent prior to taking any pictures. As you can see, even without taking items that you might be selling, the basics will quickly fill up your car trunk or van.

There are considerable time commitments for LCs providing home visits. Depending on the physical area your practice covers, you can easily spend half of your business day driving between appointments. Often, this leaves time for only two or three consults that are limited in time. If you live in a large city, traffic delays during work hours are a distinct possibility for delaying your timely arrival at a consult. Mothers and babies seen in their own home may take more time for a consult, as the telephone rings, the other children need to be cared for, she may want instruction in positioning for a variety of areas in her home, and more time-consuming issues may arise. There have been occasions when a home consultation has been scheduled, double-checked with the mother on the morning of the visit, and then no one is home when you arrive. That is time that could have been productive with another consult or back in your office with paperwork. Consider a prepayment prior to the consult or a no-show/no-cancelation fee for times such as these. Care should also be taken not to schedule consults too close together, time-wise. Consults may be much more complicated when you arrive and fully assess the situation or the mother may have many more questions than usual. Allow a cushion of time between consults for travel, traffic, complications, and emergencies.

Fees for home consultations should take into account the time spent in the home, the time spent traveling, gas and mileage on your vehicle, business insurance on your vehicle, and the payment climate in your area. Some LCs may charge a flat rate fee with a set time limit; for example, $125 for two hours. Others charge a per-mile fee for areas certain distances from their home office; for example, $125 for areas within 25 miles of zip code 12345, $150 for areas within 40 miles, $175 for areas outside of that distance. Take into consideration that mothers may have a difficult time getting their needs met if they are watching the minutes tick by on their clock, knowing another hour has just passed.

Many of your home visit costs can be written off at tax time. Take, for example, your vehicle. The Actual Expense Method allows the taxpayer to write off actual out-of-pocket costs plus depreciation if she owns the car. Examples of expenses include depreciation, licenses, tires, loan interest, road tolls, gas, oil, towing, insurance, parking fees, registration fees, lease fees, repairs, and garage rent. Keep in mind that parking and traffic tickets are not deductible. Also, if the car is used both for personal and business needs, then a percentage of use needs to be determined and the business percentage is what the owner uses for the business write-off. An example of figuring this percentage is to take your mileage reading on the morning of January 1st and the night of December 31st. Keep a mileage log for every home visit or business trip, beginning and ending figures. At the end of the calendar year, you will have total mileage driven (December 31's reading minus January 1's reading) and total mileage driven for business.

If you opt for the Standard Mileage Deduction, then track the business mileage and multiply that by the current IRS rate; the total is the deduction. In 2014, the standard mileage deduction rate is 56 cents for business miles driven, 23.5 cents for medical or moving purposes, and 14 cents in service of charitable organization. To track you might use a mileage log or a smartphone app. An example of a business mileage log includes: date, destination, business purpose, odometer start/stop and # of miles. Auto expenses are also tracked with the type and amount spent (i.e., tolls, parking fees).

If you purchase a new vehicle to be used at least in part for business purposes, some states will allow the deduction of state sales tax in that year. Your vehicle liability insurance can be deducted. Business meals with your accountant, CPA, lawyer, or with other healthcare professionals can be deducted. Save all receipts and mark them with date and details of the transaction.

Leased Office Space

If money were no object, every private practice lactation consultant would have a large office in prime retail space, providing great signage! However, as many LCs have discovered, money is the largest hurdle for having an outside brick-and-mortar office space.

If your decision is to pursue a space for your practice, be sure to locate and work closely with a commercial real estate tenet rep who specializes in office space. No matter the size of space you will need, look at all the options your rep presents to you. The tenet rep's job is to build a great rapport with you, learn your specific needs, and be available to you when you achieve more success and need to upgrade your office. You can be fairly certain that the rep knows the rental market better than you do at this stage.

Office space is expensive. For business success and financial reasons, you will want to stay in a chosen space for years. Do you anticipate business changes which will affect the space needs for your practice in the next five to ten years? Is the space move-in ready or will you need to invest in painting, carpet, counter space, etc.? Is your contract locking in a rental price for a set time or will it increase annually? Will your rent be lower if you sign a long-term contract? Is the space accessible to freeways and public transportation? Is there adequate parking space available for your clients, as well as others in the same complex? Do you have first right of refusal for adjoining spaces? Is there a plan for off-hours accessibility to the office for weekend or evening consultations? Is your potential office space easily accessible to new mothers who can't walk far and to those in wheelchairs or on crutches? Are there bathroom facilities within the office space or will mothers–and YOU–need to go down the hallway to wash their hands? And is there enough privacy in the area where you will be providing consults?

Leveraging a rental space contract can be difficult for some in private practice. When negotiating your rental contract, keep in mind your current and projected needs for the business. Think about the terms of the contract rather than the rate, as you want the best bang for your bucks in this deal. As a tenant, nothing is ever free! Better parking, a "free month's rent," and other so-called deals always benefit the landlord, and those freebies are built into the overall improvement fees passed on to all clients in that building or complex. Prior to signing your name on the dotted line, work with your real estate lawyer to thoroughly review the lease contract. Remember the tenet rep gets paid on commission, so the rep benefits if you sign the deal. You want a non-biased expert to review and assist with negotiations if needed. The lawyer gets paid regardless of the outcome. Finally, be sure to negotiate for an unexpected exit from the lease.

Shared Office Space

There is a popular movement currently underway for small start-up businesses to share office space, called co-working, serviced office space, business centers, or executive suites. Sharing an already existing office space can provide amenities that new business owners might not be able to afford in their own space, such as furniture, technology (Internet, Wi-Fi, printers, scanners, telephone services), kitchen space, a corporate address and mail services, receptionist services, and more. This cost-effective office environment frequently offers reduced pricing on additional services, such as marketing and advertising, conference or classroom space, and signage. The typical lease for shared space is six to 12 months, with some localities offering a three-month rate.

Another type of shared office space is sub-leasing space from an existing business with excess space. In this situation, your practice could potentially rent a single office or set of offices within the larger company's space, and share kitchen, telephone, conference room, and bathroom facilities.

Shared offices can provide a synergistic marketing solution for private practice LCs. By pooling your office space with related professionals, you can enjoy the compounding synergy of building your referral base with other similar non-competing businesses. Think massage therapists, chiropractors, obstetricians, pediatricians, baby specialty stores–the possibilities are limitless.

Contracts

Primary Care Providers

One possibility for a contractual relationship was given in a 2008 study by Thurman and Allen. The use of IBCLC services was integrated into a primary care practice, which was then promoted as being "breastfeeding supportive." The IBCLC was brought on as a clinic staff member who could be summoned to assist with the immediate needs of infants and/or mothers. She also provided scheduled prenatal and breastfeeding classes, follow-up appointments, and staff education.

WIC

The Women, Infants, and Children's Program (WIC) has federal funding set aside specifically for breastfeeding education, services, and promotion. Information at the USDA website reports for fiscal year 2013 that 2,046,627 pregnant, postpartum, and breastfeeding women participated in the WIC program. Participants who were breastfeeding totaled 595,318, with 249,520 fully breastfeeding and 345,798 partially breastfeeding (USDA,

2014). The Healthy, Hunger-Free Kids Act of 2010, Public Law 111-296, requires the Department of Agriculture to annually compile and publish breastfeeding performance measurements. The full results of the data report for fiscal year 2013 can be downloaded at the USDA website. Figures are available by region, state, county, city, and specific agency.

Many WIC agencies hire IBCLC services on a contract basis for client consults, staff education, and research. The Breastfeeding Coordinator for the agency can be contacted for discussion of possible contract work, and many IBCLCs write their own provision of services via clinic consults or home visits, as well as Peer Counselor trainings and staff education. The fees set are often lower than normal LC consult fees; however, your clientele are in need of quality lactation care and may not meet the criteria for other lactation programs. Paying for services is often not an option for these mothers.

Doctors, Hospitals, Birthing Centers, Home Health, Public Health…

Think outside the standard box when contemplating a contract work situation. Opportunities have been found through OB/Gyn, pediatric, and family practice offices; in a hospital; with a midwife-staffed birthing center; with doula groups; with home health services; in public health clinics; with various corporations as an expansion of the Mother Friendly Workplace services; with insurance companies; as a skilled medical provider/durable medical equipment company; with established retail centers for mother/infant products; as a speaker for educational workshops and conferences; as an expert witness for court cases; along with various other situations. Be creative and invent a new niche for your practice!

Telehealth and Online Consulting

Telehealth is a telecommunications capability that allows patients to consult with their care providers via two-way video, text, or e-mail. "Worldwide revenue for telehealth devices and services is expected to swell to $4.5 billion in 2018, up from $440.6 million in 2013," based on data from an IHS report entitled *World Market for Telehealth–2014 Edition*. The number of patients using telehealth services will rise to seven million in 2018, up from less than 350,000 in 2013" (IHS, 2014). In telehealth, electronic communication occurs over a HIPAA-compliant online connection to maintain confidentiality. An e-visit includes the total interchange of online inquiries and other communications associated with this single client encounter, and appropriate documentation is performed and maintained. The client must initiate the process and agree to e-visit service terms, the privacy policy, and fees for receiving care from the LC.

The University of Texas Health, Houston WIC department is currently using telehealth successfully in their program. Video conferencing was selected as the technology to provide distance IBCLC lactation care. Alisa Sanders says, "Our IBCLC is located in a centrally located breastfeeding support center. The local WIC clinics are located in areas that are typically geographically close to the mothers' homes. Our clients visit their local WIC offices for the consult. The mothers are never left alone during the consult. They are assisted by a remote site assistant under the direction of the IBCLC via webcam. The remote site assistant can be a peer counselor, nutritionist, or dietitian. They help the mother with positioning and operate the camera for diagnostic viewing" (Macnab, Rojjanasrirat, & Sanders, 2012).

Use of a HIPAA-compliant online service is vital to assure client confidentiality and compliance with the law. Skype states that their data is encrypted. However, according to the American Psychological Association, "liability for failure to comply with HIPAA is now shared equally by covered entities and business associates–third parties that provide services to covered entities and may have access to PHI. So it is critical for practitioners to have business associate agreements in place. Yet Skype does not offer business associate agreements for healthcare professionals who want to use it for telehealth purposes. In fact, Microsoft, which owns Skype, did not mention Skype in its April 2013 press release announcing its updated business associate agreement for its cloud services." They go on to say, "Further, Security Rule compliance requires that covered entities use technologies that include audit controls, which are mechanisms for monitoring who is accessing ePHI, as well as Breach notification tools, which are means of alerting users when there is an unauthorized disclosure of or access to ePHI. Health practitioners using Skype to communicate with clients need to be aware that, although Skype is encrypted, it is not necessarily HIPAA compliant." In the U.S., practitioners need to engage in a HIPAA Business Associate Agreement with the third party providing the online services, and that third party must be HIPAA compliant. Worth studying is a 2011 research article by Eysenbech that found passwords used to protect ePHI were hacked in 14 out of 15 of the zip files studied. "Among these, 13 files contained thousands of records with sensitive health information...and the programs which contained PHI included Microsoft Word, Microsoft Excel, SAS, and SM." Eysenbach goes on to recommend that "protocols be employed to securely exchange information using PGP (PrettyGood Privacy) or S/MME (Secure Multipurpose Internet Mail Extensions)."

Google+ has just released an option for HIPAA compliance. Google Apps can provide transmitting and storage services for private health information. However, Google Hangouts cannot provide this capability. If you desire to see and talk live with your client, you must sign a Business Associate Agreement (BAA) with Google, promising not to use Hangouts for this purpose. The BAA covers Gmail, Google Calendar, Google Drive, and Google Apps Vault. The company has just made available Helpout for Providers, which will allow a type of encryption and protect the live conversation. Scheduling is simple and handled right from Helpouts. You must set up a Google+ account, apply for an invitation code, set up a Google Wallet Merchant account, and create a Helpouts listing. Visit the Google+ Provider Hub for resources to assist in your setup.

Services that would meet the criteria for privacy can be found through Vsee. com, eprotex.com, protiviti.com, onlinetech.com, windstreambusiness. com, citrixonline.com, RSAsecurity.com, and many others. You need to research your options and shop around to get the best coverage for the best price.

Experienced LCs Share

Please describe your practice (home visits, office visits, telehealth, partner).

Having a partner in the business was mentioned by several IBCLCs, but both reported these relationships did not work well.

Many solo practitioners do have backup coverage for their practice when ill, meeting family needs, or on vacation.

None of these IBCLCs provide any type of telehealth or consulting through the Internet, nor do they provide email consultations.

Two work out of a pediatrician's office to provide services to the physician's patients, as well as having a private office in the practice.

Contracts to provide lactation services were written with WIC (Women, Infants, and Children's Program) and with hospitals.

Three LCs provide professional speaking services locally, nationally, and internationally, and one IBCLC provides intern instruction.

Only one LC provides telephone counseling, without charge, but only to existing clientele.

Over half of these solo practitioners provide home visits for consultations, with several of them mentioning a transition to only office visits because of the vast quantities of time consumed in travel to and from homes and the extremely long time spent in home consults.

Half of these IBCLCs have some sort of office space for client consultations, with several having a formal office in their own home.

Storage Requirements to Consider

Patient Records

Wherever you practice, you need to consider storage requirements. In some states, there are laws that require you to keep the consultation charting for a certain period of time. For example, some hospitals are required to keep adult records for 22 years past the last visit. When working with infants, charting for some private practice lactation consultants must be kept for 21 years or until the infant reaches "legal" age of consent. If your practice sees five consults per week, 50 weeks of the year, that is 250 individual files to keep in a water-proof, fire-proof location. Over ten years, that multiplies into 2500 files, and you can imagine the challenge of storing all that paperwork.

Do you have room in your home for all these files? If you rent office space, is there room for storage? Many private practice lactation consultants rent storage space in a climate-controlled, fire-proof storage business to keep these records. That is a monthly cost you must consider when planning your business budget. Other LCs have designed online storage systems to keep these records. Consider, though, how quickly technology changes and how you are going to access those online files in 10, 15, or 20 years.

Business Records

The storage laws for receipts of sales transactions, correspondence, legal documents, accounting records, as well as tax paperwork vary from state to state. Certain paperwork laws are federally mandated. These are excellent questions to ask your lawyer and business accountant. Smith, Koelling, Dykstr, and Ohm, certified public accountants and advisors (www.skdocpa. com/Record-Retention.htm#b1), give excellent guidelines; however, be sure to check your city, county, and state regulations to be sure you are keeping track of everything you might need. They suggest the following business documents be kept for one year: correspondence with customers and vendors, duplicate deposit slips, purchase orders, records of goods received, requisitions, notebooks (e.g., telephone calls, minutes, etc.), and stockroom withdrawal forms.

Documents to be kept for three years include bank statements and reconciliations, employee personnel records after termination, employment applications, expired insurance policies, general correspondence, internal audit reports, internal reports, petty cash vouchers, physical inventory records, savings bond registration records for employees, and time cards for hourly employees.

Six years of storage is recommended for accident reports or claims; accounts payable ledgers and schedules; accounts receivable ledgers and schedules; cancelled checks; cancelled stock and bond certificates; employment tax records; expense analysis and expense distribution schedules; expired contracts and leases; inventories of products, materials, and supplies; invoices to customers; payroll records and summaries, including payment to pensioners; copies of purchase orders; sales records; time logs; travel and entertainment records; and vouchers for payments to vendors, employees, etc.

Documents which should be kept forever include: audit reports from CPAs or accountants; cancelled checks for important payments (e.g., tax payments); cash books, chart of accounts; contracts and leases currently in effect; corporate documents (i.e., incorporation, charter, by-laws, etc.); documents substantiating fixed asset additions; deeds; depreciation schedules; financial end-of-year statements; general and private ledgers, year-end trial balance; insurance records, current accident reports, claims, policies; IRS revenue agents' reports; legal records, correspondence, and other important matters; minutes of directors and stockholders meetings; mortgages, bills of sale; property appraisals by outside appraisers; property records; retirement and pension records; tax returns and worksheets; and trademark and patent registrations.

That's a lot of information that needs to be stored!

Private Practice Self-Check

What type of office do you plan to have–home-based, home visit, or leased office space?

Will you try to contract with a primary care provider, WIC, hospital, or birthing center?

Will you provide telehealth or online consulting?

Where will you store patient and business records?

Chapter Six. Accounting Decisions

If you're not making mistakes, then you're not doing anything. I'm positive that a doer makes mistakes.

-John Wooden

There are no accounting classes required for lactation consultant certification courses. And yet this is the most important part of your business practices. The Internal Revenue Service (IRS) provides multiple publications dealing with your accounting practices, which are available for free download at www.irs.gov.

Accounting Method

The IRS requires that you figure your taxable income and file an income tax return for an annual accounting period (tax year), and that you consistently use an accounting method that clearly shows your income and expenses for the tax year. This tax year could be the calendar year or a fiscal tax year of 12 consecutive months ending on the last day of any month except December. If you filed your first income tax return using the calendar tax year and you later begin business as a sole proprietor, you must continue to use the calendar tax year unless you get IRS approval to change. This approval requires the filing of Form 1128, Application to Adopt, Change, or Retain a Tax Year, with an additional fee.

For your practice, you must choose an accounting method-a set of rules used to determine when and how income and expenses are reported. Your accounting method includes not only the overall method of accounting you use, but also the accounting treatment for any material items. The choice you make will be indicated on your first income tax return that includes a Schedule C for the business. If you desire to change your accounting method after that, you must obtain IRS approval.

The methods include:

> **The cash method:** All income and expenses are reported in the tax year they are incurred. This is the method chosen by most individuals and sole proprietors with no inventory. Qualifying taxpayers or small businesses earning under $1 million or less, or if your business is not a tax shelter as defined under section 448(d)(3) of the IRS Code, can use the cash method of accounting.

The accrual method: Matches income and expenses to the year incurred. The IRS generally requires you to use an accrual method if you produce, purchase, or sell merchandise and keep an inventory in your business.

Regardless of the accounting method chosen, you will want to have some basic accounting transactions that are kept current. A general ledger to sum up all your business transactions and sub-ledgers for accounts receivable, inventory, fixed assets, accounts payable, and payroll will get you started.

Accounts receivable keeps track of what monies are owed to your business, when it is due, and lists each customer. **Accounts payable** shows to whom you owe money and when it is due. Tracking inventory in a timely manner can provide you with information on which items sell well, when to reorder, the specialized needs of repeat clients, minimum inventory needed to meet daily sales, and material costs associated with each item.

Fixed assets are items that are for long-term use, usually five or more years, and include items such as vehicles, land, buildings, machinery, furniture and equipment. These items are not recorded when they are purchased, but rather as expenses over a period of time that coincides with their useful life. This is known as **depreciation** and is set up on a schedule. Your Certified Public Accountant (CPA) can advise you on the correct depreciation schedules for each fixed asset.

Payroll can be complicated. There are many federal and state laws regulating the items you must track related to payroll. Failure to comply can result in heavy fines or worse. Many small business owners use an outside payroll service or purchase an automated payroll software system.

Is it more affordable, both time and mistake-wise, to hire an accountant? An accountant can analyze the financial situation of your practice, offer strategic advice, produce key financial documents, serve as your outsourced chief financial officer, and file all the appropriate tax forms on time. According to Eileen P. Gunn (2011), "The typical small business can outsource its chief financial officer and accounting until the revenues rise well above the $1 million mark or until it has about 30 employees. Until then, most businesses usually don't have enough work to keep a full-time accountant busy every day."

Accounting Mistakes

In a wonderful blog on accounting mistakes that put your small business at risk (Zweig, Stepanchuk, Swyter, Smith, & Di Lauro, 2013), Josh Zweig says the number one mistake is not staying on top of receivables. This can result in hours of time wasted updating the accounts receivable, overpaying taxes, and high bad debts, resulting in loss of income for the business.

Iryna Stepanchuk says mistake number two is not keeping your expense receipts. Save a receipt of every business purchase and only use your business bank account or credit/debit card to pay business expenses.

Helena Swyter says mistake number three is not recording cash expenses. Develop a method for tracking cash expenses, as these are easily overlooked or forgotten.

Carrie Smith says mistake number four is not hiring a professional to handle the taxes. You may not claim all the deductions for which you qualify, you might underpay your tax bill, or you may not be up-to-date on the latest tax laws.

Michael Di Lauro says mistake number five is not getting on the same wavelength as your accountant. Ask your accountant to use "plain English" when discussing your account.

Accounting Software

Having high quality accounting software for your practice is important. There are many to choose from, with prices ranging from free to varying costs. Some general features are common to many:

- General ledgers to connect all accounts and support tax documenting, check handling, deposits, and payments.

- Double-entry bookkeeping that tracks where money is coming from and being spent.

- Point of sale capability to process sales, check payments, and ecommerce, such as credit cards, online purchases, and PayPal.

- Inventory management that can be linked to the point of sale feature to automatically keep track of inventory.

- Software as a Service (SaaS) which is available exclusively online.

The top rated accounting software programs include Peachtree, Xtuple Postbooks, Intuit Quickbooks and Quickbooks Online, Freshbooks, Outright, Bookkeeper, SQL-Ledger, GNU Cash, and Nola Pro (Wilson, 2010; Stevens, 2014).

Accepting credit or debit cards through your business is almost a necessity in this day and age. According to the Small Business Administration, businesses that do not accept credit cards are missing out on increasing their sales, since these cards are not only the most common method of payment, but also the most convenient. To accept cards as payment, you have multiple options for use in your practice.

Account Services

Merchant account services, such as Flagship Merchant Services, Merchant Warehouse, and National Bankcard, provide a holding location for the credit card payments your business receives. When the funds have been approved, the merchant services provider transfers the money, minus its commission, to your bank account. The needed equipment to accept debit and credit cards (POS terminals, swipers, PIN-pad terminals, wireless terminals) are provided by rental or purchase to the business as part of the merchant services. Fees are incurred with these types of services, including a monthly statement fee, a monthly minimum fee, and transaction fees, usually a percentage of the transaction and a 20+ cent fee per transaction.

Mobile card processing through Flagship ROAMpay Merchant Services, CreditCardProcessing.com, or Leaders Merchant Services is a good option for those private practitioners always on the go and who accept payments outside of their office location. It is set up to use your iPhone, iPad, smart phone, or tablet to process payments, with a card reader that plugs directly into your device to work with the app from the provider. Again, there are monthly statement fees, monthly minimum fees, and transaction fees in percentage and per transaction.

Those small business owners not wanting to deal with merchant services providers can obtain online credit card processing through PayPal, Square, GoEmerchant, EPX, or Google Checkout. These third-party providers usually have lower setup and monthly fees, but the transaction fees are typically higher than with merchant services providers. Several disadvantages might make you think hard about choosing this method. There is an increased chance of a customer disputing the charge, since the name of the third-party processor (not your practice) shows up on their monthly statement. Many customers are rerouted to the website for the processor, which increases the steps and dissuades a client from continuing with their purchase.

Pricing Your Practice Fees

There are a variety of components that factor into whether your practice will be profitable or not, including location, leadership, market demand, competition, etc. One of the more important decisions you need to make for your practice is how to price your services and products. Pricing services is often more challenging than pricing products, since you can pinpoint the cost of providing a physical product. It is more difficult to calculate the worth of your experience, knowledge, counseling, expertise, and time. And the method used to set the prices for a private lactation practice in New York City will be very different from one in small-town Texas or in a country outside of the U.S.

Inc.com suggests several considerations when developing your price structure (Wasserman, 2009):

- **Cost-plus pricing:** This method determines the cost of providing a service and then adds an additional amount to represent the desired profit. Look at your direct costs, indirect costs, and fixed costs. Consider the inclusion of a portion of your rent, utilities, transportation (vehicle, gas), rental equipment (scale, pumps), administrative costs (liability insurance, paperwork time), and general overhead costs.

- **Competitors' pricing:** You need to be aware of what competitors in your locale are charging for similar services. Gather this information from websites, phone calls, others who have used the competitor's services, published data, and competitor's written materials. Be careful about competing on prices and underpricing your own services. It is better to compete on service, reputation, ambiance, or other factors that set your practice apart from all the others. Win a client over with service, not price. You are seeking to establish long-term relationships with clients and increase your reputation and standing in the community.

- **Perceived value to the client:** Subjectivity is required here, since to your clients the important factor in determining how much they are willing to pay for your service may not be how much time you spent providing those services. Ultimately, it is the perceived value of that service and your expertise in providing it to the client that determines what you are worth. Pricing in this method becomes an art form.

In order to calculate your costs in providing a service, the U.S. Small Business Administration recommends that you include three factors: (1) material cost, (2) labor cost, and (3) overhead costs (Beesley, 2012). LCs in private practice need to figure in costs for rent, taxes, insurance, depreciation, advertising, office supplies, utilities, mileage, etc. when pricing their services. You may include a reasonable amount of these overhead costs billed to each service performed, either in an hourly rate or a percentage. And don't depend on last year's figures to determine your costs. Charge clients rates that cover your current costs.

Once you have put a figure to your costs for providing a service, know what your competitors are charging, and how your clients perceive the value of your service, you can decide whether to charge an hourly fee, a flat fee per service, or a negotiable fee.

Hourly Rate

For many businesses providing a service, an hourly rate is preferred. Hourly rates help to ensure return on the time invested in each client. Your rate should take into consideration your expertise and seniority (a more senior consultant will generally be paid a higher hourly rate than someone less experienced). Include travel time as an extra charge as recommended by the SBA.

Flat Rate

A lactation consultant charging a flat rate fee takes on the risk of losing money on the client. If you decide to charge X dollars for a full consultation, you might be wise to put a time cap on that consult, say two hours. A seemingly simple problem described in the booking of an appointment can easily turn into a four- or five-hour consult.

Negotiated Fee

If you choose to negotiate a fee, you need to determine whether you will practice a fixed-price policy and charge all your clientele the same amount or whether you will institute a variable priced policy, in which bargaining and negotiation sets the price for each client. Charging different prices for different clients can create ill will and potential loss of new clients. Mothers will talk to other mothers about what your practice did for them and how much you charged them. You cannot afford to lose integrity and respect among clients.

Terms and Conditions

Setting out your terms and conditions, along with your pricing, can prevent late payments, spending money and time on debt collection, and putting yourself at risk of uncertainty and misunderstanding, which can lead to loss of business. Your terms and conditions should be applied across all clients and include a clear definition of what products or services will be provided. Communicating payment terms and when payment is due is vital. Specifications of what happens if either party does not deliver or pay or wants to end the relationship should also be included. Keep your terms and conditions applicable to your particular business. Consult a lawyer if needed and avoid the temptation to copy another business's terms. A good source for basic contracts, templates, agreements, and terms and conditions is clickdocs.com. There you can choose from free legal documents or buy low-cost employment and business documents, financial agreements, terms and conditions, contracts, and more.

Review of Financial Statements

Regular review of your financial statements will give you feedback on whether your pricing is providing a profit (or lack of it) to your practice. Be sure to continually test new prices, new offers, and new combinations of services to help ensure increased sales. Often the perfect time to do this is when you are quoting a price to a new client. You can raise the price and offer a new, unique bonus or special service for the customer. And then track the increase or decrease in the volume of services you sell, as well as the total gross profit dollars generated by this new change. If your competition has increased their prices, consider it a good signal that the market can and will support a price increase for your services. If your clients are continually telling you what a bargain your services are, it may indicate you are charging too little for what you do. When you do raise prices, do so in small increments for each service you provide, scheduled out over the course of a period of time, say one year. Remember that you owe it to yourself and your practice to carefully manage your pricing strategy; it could mean the success or failure of your business.

Where does all the money go?

In the excitement of opening a new practice, it can be easy to get caught up in the hype of "needing this" in your practice. Whether it is a new computer program, a new computer, a copier, attending every conference available, paying for all your continuing education from the business budget, paying for credit card swipers, launching a radio ad (the pitch was too convincing!), adding a separate fax phone line, buying in bulk for a new product you're just sure every new mother will want, or whatever that expense might be, EVERYONE WANTS YOUR MONEY! Including, of course, you!

Emergency Fund

It is next to impossible to budget for every potential need and expense for your new practice. Anticipating expenses is ideal and setting aside funding for emergencies is wise. As the business owner, only you can determine what constitutes an emergency need, but this fund is the last place you should dip into for those unanticipated expenses that leave you short a few dollars. One suggestion by another practitioner is to place emergency funds into a different bank account or even a different bank than that normally used in your accounting procedure. "Hiding" these funds make it easier to resist the temptation to spend them.

Cut back in other areas of your budget if you plan to buy new equipment, find yourself having to make unexpected repairs, or dive into a new marketing venture. If you are following your budget plan, you will find the means to accomplish this task. You might also find another way to provide extra funding in the practice. Is it time you reevaluated your pricing? Can you teach classes in your office or in another local business? Is partnering with another small business owner a possibility to increase income for both of you?

Bartering

Bartering is a legal and optional method of business for private practitioners. Estimated to be a $12 billion industry in the U.S., bartering is the exchange of goods and services for other goods and services of equal value with little to no cash involvement. Small businesses can exchange almost any imaginable product or service to obtain what is needed. Medical services, media, landscaping, clothing, food, real estate, legal services, accounting services, advertising, and much more can be bartered. Advantages include receiving goods or services needed by the business without paying cash, receiving full retail value for what you are trading, utilization of time and effort, potential for new clients from the business with whom you bartered, and a better capital bottom-line for your business.

How do you go about bartering? Hundreds of barter exchange networks operate in the U.S. and can be found online with a quick engine search. The exchanges offer trade credits and can assist companies to provide services for trade credits, which then can be exchanged for another provider's services. Most exchange networks charge a fee for membership and an additional percentage fee for their exchange services. These are profit-driven associations, so be sure to compare group benefits, membership costs, and fees, and obtain member references. Check with the Better Business Bureau to obtain further information on each association.

If you barter your services privately with another company, be aware of financially troubled companies; you might never receive your portion of the barter. Attach a time and/or money value to the barter to establish a win-win situation with the other business. Your exchange should have a quantifiable equality. Assess the value of the barter to your company, making sure it will benefit you and improve your cash flow and profits.

Bartering does not offer a tax loophole to avoid taxation on the dollar amount. According to the IRS, income from bartering is taxable in the year in which you receive the goods or services. Generally, you will report this income on Schedule C, Profit or Loss from Business, Form 1040 (IRS, 2014).

Experienced LCs Share

How long were you in practice before you began drawing a paycheck for yourself?

Surprisingly, half of the practitioners are not drawing a regular paycheck for themselves. Several reported writing themselves paychecks from the very first month.

One IBCLC commented, "If I had included income for me, I would make $30 per visit which was consistently 1.5 hours clinical time and another 30-45 minutes to prepare healthcare provider reports and email the mother with an overview of her visit with attachments. This would be less than minimum wage, but expenses were covered."

One IBCLC commented on not drawing a paycheck per se, but covering all conference costs to gain CERPs, buying the needed updates in lactation textbooks, and purchasing teaching equipment, all of which are tax-deductible items.

Several other LCs took two to four years to begin drawing any type of paycheck, usually because of the ebb and flow of clients or not working at the practice a full 40 hours per week.

Having started out with paychecks when equipment rentals were lucrative, but having to back off when they dropped rentals from the practice was mentioned by several IBCLCs.

Reinvestment of any profits back into the business was frequently mentioned.

Insurance Reimbursement

The decision to apply for insurance reimbursement is a complicated one, and one that each individual practitioner must make for herself. Insurance regulations change on a frequent basis. Most companies have entire departments relegated solely to filing for insurance reimbursement.

You will need a National Provider Identifier (NPI). The Administrative Simplification provisions of the *Health Insurance Portability and Accountability Act of 1996 (HIPAA)* mandated the adoption of standard unique identifiers for healthcare providers and health plans. The purpose of these provisions is to improve the efficiency and effectiveness of the electronic transmission of health information. The Centers for Medicare & Medicaid Services (CMS) has developed the National Plan and Provider Enumeration System (NPPES) to assign these unique identifiers. Applications can be found online at the NPPES website (DHHS, 2014).

On March 31, 2014, the U.S. Senate voted 64-35 in favor of HR4032. This legislation includes language to postpone the implementation of ICD-10-CM and ICD-10-PCS until October 1, 2015. The legislation received ratification from President Obama on April 1, 2014. The main thing to note is that the transition from ICD-9-CM to ICD-10-CM/PCS will happen in 2015, not 2014 as initially planned.

For each ICD-10-CM/PCS code, the order file provides a unique five-digit "order number." The codes are numbered in "tabular order," i.e., the order in which the contents of the code system are displayed in the official document containing the system. There are over 84,000 separate codes for reimbursement (www.cms.gov). For most private practice LCs, this is an intimidating process, and one wrong code can mean no payment for your services. Therefore, the majority of LCs charge the client for the services provided and have the client seek reimbursement directly from their insurance company. One IBCLC, Pat Lindsey (2014), has developed an appropriately coded superbill for lactation consultants, which can be personalized to your practice (www.patlc.com/LVR).

For further details on reimbursement for IBCLC practices, see the article by Judith Gutowski (2012) at the USLCA website. There you will also find a presentation on The Health Care Provider Taxonomy, as well as suggested billing codes for IBCLCs.

Private Practice Self-Check

Will you use a cash or accrual method of accounting?

What type of accounting software will you use?

What type of merchant account service will you use?

How will you price your practice fees?

What terms and conditions will you provide to clients?

How will you provide them?

How often do you plan to review your financial statements?

Will you file insurance claims or let clients file their own claims?

What are some expected or unexpected expenses you might need to include in your budget?

How much do you think you will be able to set aside for an emergency fund?

What services could you barter?

Chapter Seven. Do I Carry Products or Not?

As a small businessperson, you have no greater leverage than the truth.

~John Greenleaf Whittier

Years ago, most private practice lactation consultants carried breast pumps for rent and sale; nursing wear, such as bras and clothing; nipple shields; breast shells; supplemental feeding devices; bottles which were thought to promote breastfeeding; baby slings; books; and other products that provided additional income to consult fees. For most LCs, it was these products that paid the monthly bills. However, times have changed. Researchers are giving us more information on what products are effective, and ethical and moral issues are arising more frequently.

Ethical and Moral Issues

There are key ethical principles commonly used when the provision of healthcare presents a moral dilemma. In the nursing and medical profession, the principles of nonmaleficence, beneficence, autonomy, fidelity, justice, and paternalism in the professional-patient relationship are frequently used.

Taken from the Latin adage, primum non nocere (first do no harm), the **principle of nonmaleficence** emphasizes the concept of avoidance of harm or hurt. As many treatments involve some degree of harm (pain, for example), the principle of nonmaleficence would imply that the harm should not be disproportionate to the benefit of the treatment. Working hand-in-hand with this is the **principle of beneficence**, or the desire to do good and to be compassionate, taking positive action to help others. Lactation consultants operate under these two principles on a daily basis.

The use of loyalty, fairness, truthfulness, advocacy, and dedication to clients defines the **principle of fidelity**. It involves an agreement to keep our promises and is based on the virtue of caring.

The **principle of justice** ensures a fair distribution of goods and services, along with a fair distribution of burdens and responsibilities. It also provides compensation if harm is done. Dilemmas related to justice often involve an economic or political aspect, making them difficult to contend with since the root cause lies in social injustice. The *International Code of Marketing of Breast-Milk Substitutes* is a prime example of an ideal for social justice.

Healthcare professionals frequently make decisions about diagnosis, therapy, and prognosis for their clients. Based on clinical knowledge and skills, the professional may believe that withholding or revealing certain information to the client is in their best interest. This **principle of paternalism** has been defined as "interference with a person's liberty of action justified by reason referring exclusively to the welfare . . . of the person being coerced" (Dworkin, 1988). This principle denies people the right to choose their own ends of action, breaching the client trust of the provider.

The **principle of autonomy** is the personal rule of the self that is free from both controlling interferences by others and from personal limitations that prevent meaningful choice. Autonomous individuals act intentionally, with understanding and without controlling influences. This is true informed consent–provision of all the positive and negative effects, information, and research–and allowing the client to make the best decision for their situation.

A **conflict of interest** is anything that impedes or might be perceived to impede an individual's or practice's ability to act impartially and in the best interest of a client. Conflicts of interest arise when the professional responsibilities of individuals or businesses are, or have the potential to be, compromised by other external obligations. A good example that is plaguing the lactation community right now is whether a lactation consultant in private practice should carry pumps and equipment for sale to increase business profits. As healthcare providers, LCs are to provide the best in evidence-based care to their clients and should be marketing good healthcare for mothers and babies. Conflict of interest arises when we appear to push product use on a client "in her best interest." Is it truly in HER best interest or in the best interest of your practice? You decide.

These principles need to be considered when deciding if, and what, products could be carried in your private practice. IBCLCs are required to adhere to the *Standards of Practice for International Board Certified Lactation Consultants* (ILCA, 2013), including practicing within the scope of the *International Code of Marketing of Breast-Milk Substitutes* and all subsequent World Health Assembly resolutions. They are also to "remain free of conflict of interest," "disclose any financial or other conflicts of interest," and "maintain an awareness of conflict of interest in all aspects of work, especially when profiting from the rental or sale of breastfeeding equipment and services." Lactation consultants must work to provide breastfeeding care with the mother and infant's best interests in mind.

"The Code"

What is the World Health Organization/UNICEF *International Code of Marketing of Breast-Milk Substitutes* (The Code; WHO, 1981)? Adopted as a recommendation in May, 1981, The Code serves to "contribute to the provision of safe and adequate nutrition for infants, by the protection and promotion of breast-feeding, and by ensuring the proper use of breast-milk substitutes, when these are necessary, on the basis of adequate information and through appropriate marketing and distribution." Since it is a recommendation, it is not legally binding for WHO Member States, although they are expected to adhere to the aim and spirit of The Code. The United States is the only member country to vote against the adoption of The Code. In the *2011 Status Report on Country Implementation of the International Code of Marketing of Breast-Milk Substitutes*, WHO reports on the status of The Code in 199 countries around the globe. Of those, only 69 countries have fully implemented it into law, with many of those countries implementing it only partially. This 50 page report can be downloaded free of charge from the WHO website.

How does The Code affect you as a private practice lactation consultant? Consider what the 14 provisions cover and how that impacts your carrying products:

1. No advertising of products under the scope of The Code to the public. These products include breastmilk substitutes, such as formula, follow-on formula, other milk products, and any food or beverage that is used as a partial or full replacement for breastmilk, as well as feeding bottles and teats (nipples). If you carry a particular brand of bottle for sale because you believe it to be the best one to use for breastfeeding infants, it cannot be advertised or on display to the public.

2. No free samples to mothers. If you carry an emergency stash of formula for those infants who must be fed immediately, what do you carry? And do you give any unopened containers to the mother to take home "for the next feeding"? Think about it...

3. No promotion of products in healthcare facilities, including the distribution of free to low-cost supplies. No Code-breaking freebies of any kind should enter your practice. Period.

4. No company representatives to advise mothers. Some IBCLCs choose not to carry products from non-Code compliant companies. As a business professional who abides by a Code of Ethics and Code of Conduct, you will need to make a decision regarding these companies. The "lactation experts" provided by these non-Code compliant companies usually have a hidden agenda, i.e., they are sales personnel for that company. Their ultimate goal is not exclusive breastfeeding.

5. No gifts or personal samples to healthcare workers. ANY non-Code compliant company who tries to provide your practice with samples and freebies should be turned down.

6. No words or pictures idealizing artificial feeding, including pictures of infants, on the labels of the products. How many nipple companies have you seen with wording that implies

their product is better for breastfeeding? How about photos of a happy baby being bottle-fed? Think about it, if you carry a product that falls under The Code, does it contain words or pictures idealizing anything else but breastfeeding?

7. Information to health workers should be scientific and factual. And it should be unbiased. Who pays for the research? Who provides the products for the research? How is the research done, and how does the wording in the conclusion support or negate breastfeeding?

8. All information on artificial feeding, including the labels, should explain the benefits of breastfeeding and all costs and hazards associated with artificial feeding. Many labels currently on products do not provide this information.

9. Unsuitable products, such as sweetened condensed milk, should not be promoted for babies.

10. All products should be of a high quality and take into account the climatic and storage conditions of the country where they are used.

11. Promote and support exclusive breastfeeding for six months as a global public health recommendation with continued breastfeeding for up to two years of age and beyond.

12. Foster appropriate complementary feeding from the age of six months, recognizing that any food or drink given before nutritionally required may interfere with breastfeeding.

13. Complementary foods are not to be marketed in ways to undermine exclusive and sustained breastfeeding.

14. Financial assistance from the infant feeding industry may interfere with professionals' unequivocal support of breastfeeding. For lactation consultants, this includes "free" educational sessions, scholarships, dinners, trips to conferences, etc., and payments for speaking from non-Code compliant companies.

Breast pumps and collection/storage containers are not covered under The Code. However, if a particular product is produced by a company who violates The Code with several of their other products, do you want to carry their item in your practice? Think about your position. In becoming a "sales person," as well as a "spokesperson" for this company, you become complicit in their violation just by association with them, giving the impression of condoning the violation. If you do carry that product, it cannot be prominently displayed or marketed to mothers in your office, in advertisements, or in your visits to mothers' homes.

The WHO, International Baby Food Action Network (IBFAN),UNICEF, Save the Children, NABA, and other international organizations monitor the implementation of The Code across the world, both independently and with governments. WHO provides amendments and resolutions to The Code whenever necessary.

Due to these confusing and complicated moral and ethical issues, many private practice lactation consultants have chosen not to rent or sell products of any kind. The few products they carry are for use in consultations, such as feeding devises, nipple shields, etc. And several brands are usually carried to meet the needs of the mothers and infants, rather than promoting a particular brand.

Experienced LCs Share

Please share at least three other services you offer other than lactation consults.

All of the IBCLCs represented here provide other services to generate income in their private practice. Those mentioned include: support groups; classes for prenatal needs, breastfeeding, mothering, or childbirth; doula services; mentoring and education for newer lactation professionals (IBCLCs, La Leche League Leaders, WIC Peer Counselors); a weekly newsletter; massage appointments for infants, pregnant mothers, and postpartum mothers; specialized consults for pumping, returning to employment, and prenatally; and lectures for local hospitals and baby stores.

Not quite half of the respondents also provide retail services in the form of breast pump rentals and sales; pump parts; supplies, such as nipple shields, hand pumps, milk storage bags and trays; nipple creams; nursing bras; nursing pillows; and herbal galactogogues.

Those IBCLCs with specializations also offer additional services: Alison Hazelbaker provides craniosacral therapy and psychology process work sessions; Liz Brooks provides expert witness services for litigation involving lactation issues and ethical advice to IBCLCs; and Pat Lindsey sells a packet of business forms, including a lactation "superbill," with information on insurance reimbursement, newly revised to include the ICD-10 coding and information on the Affordable Care Act.

Choosing Products

When carrying products for use in and sale/rent by your practice, there are several areas of research that will assist you in making the best decisions for your business.

Having adequate capital to order and carry enough products is important. Many companies require a minimum wholesale order for their products, which can be a costly investment as a new practitioner. And remember that it takes time to show a profit in small business. In fact, it takes most small businesses an average of three to five years to see a profit.

Choosing which products to carry can be a daunting task. You will want to have the right merchandise on hand, at the right time, and in the right quantities to meet the needs of your clients. There should be a demand for your products in the area you wish to serve, and the competition cannot be so heavy that you have no chance of renting or selling your products. Having to compete against the budget, marketing, and advertising strategies of the big chain stores can be disheartening. But you need to have something unique in your practice, something that ONLY YOU can provide. Find that something and build on it. Your product selection does not need to appeal to everyone, but you do want to provide products that will turn a profit and be in demand by a good number of clients.

Consider these questions when deciding which products to choose:

- Does it promote, protect, and support breastfeeding?

- Would you buy it and use it yourself?

- Can you stand behind the product unquestioningly?

- Are you excited about the product and its benefits?

- Would you sell it to a close friend or family member?

- Is there a strong need for the product in the current market?

- Can you see yourself selling the product for the next several years?

- Is there any non-industry supported research on this product?

Being knowledgeable about your products is a value to bring to your practice. Don't make a product decision based on what other lactation support sales shops carry. Talk to your clientele, other LCs, and manufacturer's sales reps, read testimonials, and attend conferences and trainings where these products are discussed. You need to know about pricing structure, various models available, the history of the product, details on use of the product, common complaints, and the manufacturer's servicing, warranty, and repair policies. Knowing the product inside and out will allow excellent service, education, and assistance to the mothers with whom you work.

No matter the product, if your clients are not buying it, the profitability of your practice will decrease. Know your customers and their needs. Choose a product with recurring sales value, such as items that need to be replaced on a regular basis, as well as related items to that product. Research what is popular at the time, since new trends and products can increase your clientele. Competition is healthy; there are other means to compete for clients than pricing. The more unique your product, the more clients it will generate. And, of course, choose only high-quality products to keep building the excellence of your reputation. Appendices F, G, H, and I provide a list of companies that provide various products you might want to carry.

Inventory

Space for storing your product inventory is important, as is a method to track the inventory itself. For example, think of the size of rental breast pumps: do you have space for storing six, a dozen, two dozen pumps, especially if they are all in your inventory at once. Add space for the kits to use with each pump rental, space to store the shipping boxes they arrived in for return to the company, cleaning products and a cleaning location for the pumps, spare parts for replacing lost or damaged ones, and more. The need for space grows exponentially.

Keeping track of your inventory can be daunting. Inventory management can be described as the practice of planning, directing, and controlling inventory, so that it contributes to the profitability of your private practice and you have items to meet client needs when called for. Spreadsheets can be one inexpensive method to track a small inventory. Keep in mind, though, that data on a spreadsheet can be accidentally deleted or changes not imported into the program. Some beginning LCs keep a handwritten inventory to get the practice up-and-running. When you are very busy, though, it is too easy to forget to make written inventory changes.

Many business coaches recommend a specific inventory control program. You can start with Quickbooks or Peachtree, which include in their accounting packages an inventory feature. They can even provide a dollar value to the inventory at various points. This is especially helpful at the end of the calendar year when you must pay taxes on your current inventory. These programs also enable you to track trends and match purchase orders with inventory received, alerting you when inventory is low.

Stand-alone inventory tracking programs can also be purchased through netsuite.com, fishbowlinventory.com, epicor.com, ultriva.com, manageengine.com, oracle.com, and others.

Decisions on the amount of inventory to carry are based on three costs: ordering, holding, and shortage. Ordering costs include the time spent preparing purchase orders, finding and talking with suppliers, transportation costs (such as postage, UPS, FedEx), and time spent unpacking the inventory and storing it in your system.

Holding costs consist of the dollar amount you pay for storage space, security systems used in your practice, insurance, the amount of working capital you have tied up in inventory, and the costs of products damaged, stolen, no longer needed, or obsolete.

Shortage costs include lost revenue when your practice does not have an item, the items are on backorder, or the shipment is lost en route. It also includes the loss of credibility when this happens with regularity and loss of clients to other practices because you cannot meet their needs at that moment.

Pricing Your Products

As a retailer (remember you are carrying products for sale or rent), you are in practice to make a profit. Setting the right selling price for the items your practice carries is fundamental to seeing a profit or loss at the end of the year. It is necessary to consider the cost of the product, shipping and handling, and the cost of operating your business, including overhead, marketing and advertising costs, office supplies, etc. Whatever selling price is decided upon, it must cover all of these items. If the price is too low, you will not succeed in business. On the opposite side of the coin, if the items you carry are sold in a variety of other locations for much less, the inventory will build up in your practice, and your profit will decrease.

Many suppliers provide a suggested retail price for businesses selling their products. There are instances when the supplier will require that their product pricing does not go below this suggested pricing. It is known in lactation circles that big-box stores and some online sources sell breastfeeding products at much lower prices. This provides the private practice lactation consultant with a challenge: how to obtain clients. Once again, the emphasis becomes what can YOU and only you provide in the way of outstanding client service?

Pricing strategies which can be used in the decision-making process can include pricing below the competition; prestige pricing, which is exclusivity, location, or unique client service that can justify higher pricing; psychological pricing, using figures that end in 5, 7, or 9, giving the perception of rounding down a price of $10.95 to $10 rather than $11; keystone pricing or doubling the cost paid for the product; multiple pricing, pairing several products for one price–this is great for sales, markdowns, or reducing inventory space to add a new product; discount pricing and price reductions using coupons, rebates, or seasonal pricing; and/or loss leaders, pricing a product below its cost to increase traffic to the practice.

Increasing Sales

All small business owners will experience, at one time or another, a decline in clients, seasonal sales, or new competition in their area that causes a slump in sales or consults. How can sales be increased?

Advertise, advertise, advertise. Plan to spend a larger portion of the budgeting dollars on getting the word out about products and services offered by your practice.

Generate a buzz. Use social marketing to start lively conversations through blogging, Tweeting, or a Facebook page. Offer classes through your office or at another location. Attend networking meetings and events, such as the Chamber of Commerce, the local nursing mothers group, the lactation consultants group, new mothers groups, etc. Send a press release to your local newspaper and to television and radio stations. Offer a unique promotional event. Sponsor and attend community events. Get the name of your practice on everyone's lips!

Double-check your pricing. Are your prices too high? They should be competitive, but still profitable.

Set up. If you have a brick-and-mortar location, use display ideas that will highlight products, such as lighting, educational video demonstrations, music, aromatherapy scents, or even live entertainment.

Who is your client? Connect with the mothers, grandparents, parents, and relatives of the clients you hope to serve. Determine their needs and desires. Provide education with all the products carried in the practice. Offer added-value services, such as a referral credit. Establish a mailing list for feedback, information on new items, or suggestions from clientele.

Consider each of the topics in this chapter when you write your business plan and when compiling your policies and procedures handbook. Plenty of pre-planning and thought will benefit your private practice in the long run.

Private Practice Self-Check

Do you want to carry products?

How will you comply with the Code?

What products will you carry?

Where will you store inventory?

How will you price your products?

How will you increase sales if there is a slump?

Chapter Eight. What Else Do I Need?

Happiness lies in the joy of achievement and the thrill of creative effort.

- Franklin D. Roosevelt

Insurance Coverage

Wherever you decide to practice, you will want to look into several vital concepts prior to opening your practice. The first is insurance coverage. At a minimum, you should have malpractice insurance to cover your professional actions. Professional liability insurance (PLI), also called professional indemnity insurance or errors and omissions insurance, is a form of insurance that helps protect professional advice and services, so that the full cost of defending against negligence, misrepresentation, violation of good faith and fair dealing, or inaccurate advice brought in a lawsuit by a client does not fall on the lactation consultant. PLI coverage is generally set up based on a per-claim basis, with a specified coverage period. Each policy is different, and you will want to read policy coverage very carefully. PLI does not cover criminal prosecution or legal liability under civil law. Some policies can have added cyber liability coverage. Keeping your coverage current is important, as the protection ends the same day the policy expires. Some insurance carriers will not allow professionals to backdate a coverage policy. It is rare that a grace period is allowed on these policies.

Why liability insurance? In this time of increased consumer knowledge and awareness of their rights to full investigation for incidents, suits seeking retribution for damages or perceived damages abound. Working with mothers and infants, potential exists for accidental injury or harm to come as a result of negligent behavior or omission by the practicing lactation consultant. Even if you have the best intentions and provide your best care, an inquest, criminal court case, or civil lawsuit can follow such an incident. This means out-of-pocket expenses for you, increased stress, and damage to your professional reputation.

Malpractice insurance can be found for allied health professionals, including IBCLCs, CLCs, doulas, occupational therapists, speech language pathologists, and many others through several carriers. Rates vary according to your state, location of your practice, whether you are being covered for more than one specialty, and whether you work part-time or full-time hours. USLCA previously offered discounted rates to members, but has since discontinued this benefit of membership.

As a small business owner, a general liability insurance policy can protect your practice premises and operations, products, data breach, fire liability, medical payments for "slips and falls," vehicle use for home visits, employer liability, and employment practices. Whether you have clients come to your home-based business, you provide home visits to their home, or you have a free-standing office to provide services to clients, you will need general liability insurance. There are many companies who provide this coverage to small businesses—State Farm, Farmers, Nationwide, and Hartford—to name a few.

Vaccinations

Another vital consideration is your vaccination status. Healthcare workers are at risk for exposure to serious diseases and can act as carriers of these diseases to newborn infants and their mothers. The Centers for Disease Control and Prevention (CDC, 2013) recommends that all healthcare workers are up-to-date with the following vaccinations:

- Hepatitis B—a three-dose series of #1 now, #2 in one month, and #3 five months after #2.

- Annual Flu—a one-dose annual vaccine

- MMR (Measles, Mumps and Rubella)—If you were born in 1957 or later and have not had the MMR vaccine or if you don't have an up-to-date blood test which shows you are immune to measles, mumps, and rubella, you will need two doses of MMR four weeks apart.

- Varicella (Chickenpox)—If you have not had chickenpox, if you haven't had the varicella vaccine, or if you don't have an up-to-date blood test that shows you are immune to varicella, you will need two doses of varicella vaccine, four weeks apart.

- Tdap (Tetanus, Diphtheria, Pertussis)—If you have not received Tdap previously, you will need a one-time dose now, and a Tdap booster every ten years.

- Meningococcal—If you are regularly exposed to isolates of N. *meningitides,* you should receive one dose. You should get the meningococcal vaccine if you have a damaged spleen or your spleen has been removed, have terminal complement deficiency, *or* are traveling or residing in countries in which the disease is common.

State laws vary on immunization requirements for healthcare workers, so be sure to check your state's regulations. Any contract work done for a hospital, home healthcare provider, public health clinic, WIC clinic, or physician practice will require these basic immunizations.

Forms

As a new lactation consultant in private practice, you will be developing forms to use with your clients to document an assessment and consult, establish a plan of care, and communicate consult findings with primary care practitioners. Legal considerations in the Standards of Practice for International Board Certified Lactation Consultants (ILCA, 2013) require an explanation of applicable fees for services prior to providing care; informed consent from all clients prior to assessment, intervention, reporting relevant information to other healthcare providers, taking photographs/audio/digital/electronic recordings, and when seeking publication of information associated with a consult; documentation of an appropriate history of the breastfeeding mother and child; assessment of objective and subjective information; development of a plan of care; provision of oral and written instructions for the plan of care; follow-up strategies; and sharing of research-based, current information on breastfeeding and clinical skills.

Prepared forms for lactation charting can be ordered with your logo and practice information from Mahala Lactation and Perinatal Services, LLC, (Myler, West, & Lisimachio, 2014) or Bay Area Breastfeeding & Education, LLC, (Jolly & Ryan, 2014). The International Lactation Consultant Association website has samples of many types of lactation forms you can adapt to your practice. iTunes has a downloadable app for your iPad called Mobile Lactation Consultant, allowing a HIPAA compliant record of all patient information (health history, prior pregnancies, financial information, etc.); a record of client visits, infant exams, maternal exams, breastfeeding assessment, plan of care; a record of telephone, text, and email conversations; a customer billing tracker; task lists; appointment scheduler; CPT and ICD codes for billing insurance companies; and lock features to protect client information. This service from Mobile Lactation Consultant runs from $19 to $49 per month (Daly Enterprises, Inc., 2014). Forms can also be self-designed in programs such as jetform.com, wufoo.com, formstack.com, formsite.com, and emailmeform.com.

Lactationmatters.org recently published an article by Jessica Lang Kosa, PhD, IBCLC, on taking private practice paperless (2013). Keeping an electronic health record avoids wasted paper, saves storage space, allows integration of emails into client files, and makes communication with clients and primary care providers easier and quicker.

Appointments

Making online appointments also helps the practice go paperless and provides immediate service for mothers needing assistance. There are online scheduling programs at bookfresh.com, appointy.com, genbook.com, and checkappointments.com. These programs are compatible with Windows, Mac, smart phones and android phones. The mother can schedule the appointment online within the timelines you have set on the program using any media device.

Various lactation consultants in private practice provide their intake form on their website–available for the new client to download, complete, and return prior to her consultation. This can save a great deal of time, whether you provide home consults or see the client in your office.

Policies, Protocols, and Procedures

Developing practice policies and protocols for your private practice has several advantages. If you incorporate your business, this will be a requirement. If you have more than one person in your practice, you can use the policies and procedures as a framework for consistency and fairness. Your policies and procedures provide a direct link between your business vision and day-to-day operations. And they serve as a means to protect the legal interests of your company.

Let's start with definitions. A policy tell us what to do and why, and is a predetermined course of action established as a guide toward accepted objectives and strategies for the business. Procedures (standards, guidelines, philosophy, or rules) describe when and how, and are the methods used to carry out a policy. A treatment protocol describes in detail how a treatment should be completed based on the criteria for the lactation industry.

When developing your policies and procedures, a good starting place is with your mission statement. There are four key elements found in effective mission statements: value, inspiration, plausibility, and specificity. In a couple of short sentences, you should be able to convey the value of your company to those you serve.

From the mission statement, short objectives can be set. These are goals which direct attention to important factors in the running of your business. These factors can include customers, quality, financial performance, operations, products, marketing, and/or employees. Your policy manual should serve as a "living document," dynamic and subject to changes and updates.

Established policies and procedures ensure that your way of doing business doesn't deviate or deteriorate over time, even if staff changes. They are tailored for your business and the job, not to a specific employee. Having well-established policies and procedures can help a company refute allegations of legal or regulatory violations that employees or customers may lodge against them. They provide proof of intent, but must be accompanied by genuine efforts to adhere to federal, state, and local rules. They provide rules and guidelines for decision-making in routine situations. One example would be customer refunds. Having a written policy on refunds prevents inconsistent application of refunding, which might depend upon the client or your mood that day. The policy provides an accepted method of dealing with complaints and misunderstandings to help avoid claims of bias and favoritism.

One of your policies should address clinical documentation. The International Board of Lactation Consultant Examiners (IBLCE) defines clinical documentation as "the written, typed, or electronic record of information about a client or client group, which details the care provided. Client health records may be paper or electronic, such as electronic records, faxes, emails, audio or video recordings, as well as pictures and diagrams. The record communicates observations, assessment, plan, interventions, evaluation, outcome and follow-up. Documentation has the potential to be admitted into legal proceedings" (IBLCE, 2012). All documentation must be accurate, clear, comprehensive, and concise; contemporaneous; documented by the clinician herself; dated, timed and signed; legible and permanent; and using only accepted abbreviations to that organization and/or legal requirements.

International Board Certified Lactation Consultants are accountable for the care they provide and, therefore, their documentation of clinical events (see the Code of Professional Conduct for IBCLCs and Standards of Practice.) Mahala Lactation and Perinatal Services, LLC, has developed excellent clinical charting forms which lactation consultants can purchase and personalize with their logo and company information. The forms include two care plans, one with references and page numbers to the latest edition of *The Womanly Art of Breastfeeding;* two consent forms, one U.S. based and one for outside of the U.S.; two intake call scripts, one for home visits and one for office visits; a referral pad; a superbill; and a pump rental agreement. An update service is also available with the purchase. For more information, contact Diana West at Diana@mahalamom.com. Private practitioners Leah Jolly and Misti Ryan of Bay Area Breastfeeding & Education, LLC, have also designed forms that can be customized with your practice logo and information. Their forms include a one-page intake/history, a two-page assessment, a one-page follow-up form, a care plan, invoices, return to work form, and for the healthcare provider, a report template and introduction letter. Contact Leah and Misti at www. bayareabreastfeeding.net for more information.

Many books and online template sources can be found for writing policies and procedures. Many small business owners have found it helpful to have a copy on their computer and a binder with the full mission statement, objectives, policies, procedures, and protocols available for viewing by clients or others who might need access to it. Keeping each item to one or two pages and in individual sections makes updating the policy and procedure manual much easier, and prevents having to reprint the entire manual with each update.

Telephone Professionalism

As a private practice lactation consultant, your priority as a small business owner must be first in your mind. Keeping a separate telephone number for your practice shows professionalism to the mother who calls for breastfeeding assistance. If she hears messages about your teenagers not passing along telephone messages to you, your favorite comedian's set of one-liners, the political views you hold, or other voicemail messages commonly found on private lines, she may think twice about using your skills as a lactation consultant. Many small business professionals keep a smartphone number dedicated to their practice. Volunteers of breastfeeding counseling organizations will find this especially important, as it is difficult to separate volunteer counseling calls from professional, fee-for-service calls you might receive on the same telephone number. Make sure your voicemail message is professional and provides important information, but is not too lengthy. Let the client know when she can expect to receive a return phone call to set an appointment with you. And remember to include your website information.

Organizational Tools

Many private practice LC businesses keep the majority of their data on the computer. As your business grows, you may find this is the case for the documents, files, intake forms, research articles, healthcare provider reports, policies, and procedures you accrue over time. Keeping this information on paper requires a fire-safe, waterproof location, as well as thousands of paper files, large filing cabinets, and space—lots of it!

At www.makeuseof.com, writer Aaron Couch (2014) has provided an excellent tutorial for computer organization and management. He recommends properly and appropriately labeling folders on the computer and filing documents into those folders as they fit topically. Adding dates to each saved document can be helpful. Subfolders can be advantageous, as can jump lists, which allow you to pin folders to the Windows Explorer pop-up icon on the Taskbar. Only essential files should be on your desktop—those you access daily for example. Archive rather than delete old files and remove duplicate files.

Many busy business owners and computer users have their favorite software and organizational tools. Here are seven possible programs to assist in organization:

1. *TODOIST* features a simple and intuitive interface that helps you get organized without getting in your way. You can set due dates on your tasks and get an overview of what needs to get done today, tomorrow, or next week. It comes with a built-in calendar and alerts. Free and premium versions are available.

2. *Ta-da List* is the Internet's easiest to-do list tool. You can make lists for yourself and share them with others. You can create item lists and check them off. There is no built-in calendar. It is perfect for the list maker.

3. *EVERNOTE* allows you to easily capture information in any environment using whatever device or platform you find most convenient, and makes this information accessible and searchable at any time from anywhere. It is good for organizing information and storing ideas as they arise. You can easily categorize into "buckets" by tagging information. It works with all browsers, is free, and has a smartphone app.

4. *Backpack* is an easy intranet for your business, with the ability to store, share, discuss, and archive. It is great for time management. It offers group calendars and file sharing. There is a cost involved to download the software.

5. *Remember The Milk* manages tasks quickly and easily, with reminders to you anywhere through AIM, Skype, SMS text, and more. There are features with calendars and smart phone sync, as well as syncing with your GPS. This is a free program.

6. *Vitalist* is an online software application that categorizes tasks into specific lists or buckets. The tool is a personal organizer and productivity system, and can coordinate with your iPhone. The free version may suffice for the sole proprietor; the next level of support is $5/month.

7. *Nirvana* is all about getting things out of your head and into a trusted system, then effortlessly drilling down to the thing you should be doing right now. It will coordinate with your email account, but does not yet have a smartphone app. It is currently free.

Additional software programs that run less than $50 to purchase include AnyTime Organizer, My Ultimate Organizer, Efficient Man's Organizer, C-Organizer, LeaderTask, VIP Organizer, Exstora Pro, and MyLife Organized. All are rated as good to excellent in "Organizer Software Review 2014" by Consumers Reports.

Back Up Files

Backing up files on a regular basis is highly recommended by professionals who have lost valuable data with a computer malfunction, virus, or crash. Several options include iCloud or Dropbox, an offsite back-up location, jump or thumb drives, CD/DVDs, hard drive partitions, or a separate onsite external hard drive device. Be cautious with sensitive material, making sure it is properly encrypted and password protected. Sites such as iCloud and Dropbox are not encrypted and client information should not be stored on these sites. Backup options can be full backup, which copies all your necessary data, can require a lot of storage space, and takes a long time to save and restore if needed. Once the first full backup is completed, it is generally better to provide differential and/or incremental backups routinely. A differential backup saves files that have been changed or added since the full backup. Incremental backup saves files that have been changed or added since the last backup, either full or differential.

Consumer Reports (Snoke, 2014) lists the most highly rated data backup software programs as being NovaBACKUP, DT Utilities PC Backup, Acronis True Image, Genie Backup Manager, Macrium Reflect, Acronis Backup & Recovery, Easeus Todo Backup, NTI Backup Now, TurboBackup, and PowerBackup. All offer full, incremental, and differential backup; individual file and folder backup; network locations backup; password protection, data compression, backup verification, and create a bootable backup; restoration of files and folders, file paths, and older files and duplicates; event logs; and email support and assistance. Costs for these programs are generally below $50.00.

Private Practice Self-Check

What insurance coverage do you need?

What are the prices for the insurance in your area?

What vaccinations do you need?

What forms do you need to have when you start your practice?

How will you set up appointments?

What policies, protocols, and procedures will you need to write?

How will you make sure your phone is answered professionally?

What type of organizational tools will you use?

How will you back up your files?

Chapter Nine. Learning from the Experiences of My Peers

Alone we can do so little; together we can do so much.

~Helen Keller

Peer support, peer learning, cooperative learning, mentoring, collaborative learning: each describes researched topics from the social work, educator, medical, nursing, and professional business realms. And each is a vibrant resource for the lactation consultant in private practice to tap into. Peer learning can be defined as the acquisition of knowledge and skill through active helping and supporting among status equals or matched companions (Topping, 2005). Cooperative learning provides structured positive interdependence in the pursuit of a specific shared goal or output (Topping, 2005). Peer support functions to provide assistance in daily practice management, provide social and emotional support, share resources, and maintain extended support over time. This can be accomplished via on-line discussion groups, phone calls, text messages, meetings, and conferences, and relies on non-hierarchical, reciprocal relationships, understanding, and trust.

Peer support is crucial to private practice lactation consultants, since peers understand the environment and situation of private practice without explanation. As care providers in private practice, LCs are especially prone to loneliness and isolation. The spirit of competitiveness is rampant in many locations, barring many in private practice from sharing the joys and frustrations of their work with other lactation professionals in their local area. The fear of not being accepted, being thought of as incompetent, being betrayed, being misunderstood, or thought of as weak stops many lactation consultants from sharing with local LCs. It is essential that LCs develop attitudes that include nurturance, spirit of community, camaraderie, and trust in order to have strong alliances, networks, work teams, and peer relationships. Doing so enables them to accept and provide support to peers when needed.

Research showing how people grow and change emphasizes the importance of encouragement and reinforcement of positive decision-making. Peer support brings the unique perspective of others' stories, practical experience, and understanding, and offers empathy, knowledge of available resources, positive role modeling, and a strong sense of responsibility for others (Tunajek, 2007). The consequences of compassion fatigue, burnout, overwork, sleep deprivation, and constant change requires that professionals support, care for, and encourage each other.

Peer learning in the business world involves working with groups of like-minded individuals that want to cooperatively develop their knowledge and expertise to develop and implement new ideas based on shared experiences, ingenuity and creativity (Edlink, 2014).

Professional Women's Organizations

Let's look at a variety of sources where private practice lactation consultants and women business owners can give and receive valuable peer support. Here are some professional organizations you may want to join:

Women on Business (www.womenonbusiness.com):   Established in 2007, Women on Business is an award-winning online destination for the news and information women need to be successful in the business world from today's thought leaders. Women on Business delivers valuable information, as well as career and educational resources, to business women working in all areas of business. It was included in Forbes.com list of the Top 100 Websites for Women and the Top 20 Social Media Marketing Sites, as well as The Little Pink Book's Top 10 Business Blogs for Women.

National Association of Women Business Owners (www.nawbo. org): Founded in 1975, the National Association of Women Business Owners (NAWBO) represents America's more than 10 million women-owned businesses. NAWBO is a one-stop resource to help women business owners achieve greater economic, social, and political power.

American Business Women's Association (www.abwa.org): The mission of the American Business Women's Association (ABWA) is to bring together business women of diverse occupations and to provide opportunities for them to help themselves and others grow personally and professionally through leadership, education, networking support, and national recognition. While not a university, ABWA offers members the opportunity to participate in KU-MBA Essentials, a twelve-course program focused on the essentials of management education delivered by professors and adjunct faculty from the Kansas University School of Business.

U.S. Women's Chamber of Commerce (www.uswcc.org): The U.S. Women's Chamber of Commerce® works with and for its members to grow successful businesses and careers. The Women's Chamber supports women's business growth, retirement security, education, and employment opportunities.

Professional Business Women's Network (www.pwbn.org): The PWBN is a national, non-profit group that was established to bring together businesswomen to network and share their expertise with other businesswomen. Each chapter holds monthly meetings to enrich members' knowledge and expand their network. PWBN publishes a women's business/lifestyle magazine "About Her," featuring articles from writers who are experts in their field.

National Association of Professional Women (www.napw.com): The National Association of Professional Women (NAPW) is an exclusive network for professional women to interact, exchange ideas, educate, and empower. NAPW provides seminars, podcasts, webinars, keynote speakers, and educational tools to enable members to achieve personal and career success. NAPW supports and endorses charities and nonprofit organizations focused on women's issues and child wellness.

National Association for Moms in Business (www.momsinbusiness. org): The National Association for Moms in Business (NAFMIB) provides opportunities, education, and advocacy for moms in business to cultivate leadership, foster social justice, and develop greater economic growth potential. Moms in Business programs are available to members only, although membership is free. Moms in Business provides a variety of programs filled with tools, tips, services, and educational materials to assist in building a successful business and bringing balance to the work and life of women.

National Association of Women Owned Small Businesses (www. nawosb.webs.com): Established October 11, 2010, the National Association of Women Owned Small Businesses, Inc. (NAWOSB) has a mission to educate owners of women-owned businesses about government bids, certifications, contracts and other opportunities. Realizing most business owners do not consider or understand how to do business with the government, NAWOSB is committed to help educate, build, certify, and support companies serious about pursuing the government market.

National Association of Christian Women Entrepreneurs (www. nacwe.org): The National Association of Christian Women Entrepreneurs connects women who are ready to create, collaborate, and contribute to changing the world. Through online content, tele-courses, individual/ group coaching, and retreats, its goal is to help each member succeed and thrive in business. NACWE Membership is open to women entrepreneurs, small business owners, and others who have the desire to launch their entrepreneurial venture.

National Association of Christian Women In Business (www. nacwib.com): The National Association of Christian Women in Business (NACWIB) was founded in 2004 to equip women from around the world with the support and inspiration to gain prosperity and success in the world of business. From finding a new career, to getting a job, to starting a business on the side, NACWIB provides tools and support. The National Association of Christian Women in Business teaches women of integrity how to find success in their business operations.

The Jewish Woman Entrepreneur (www.thejwe.com): The Jewish Woman Entrepreneur (The JWE) is a national educational nonprofit organization with the mission to promote financial stability and independence among Jewish Women business owners by offering access to business education, professional training, and financial support.

Female Entrepreneur Association International (www.female entrepreneurassociation.com): The Female Entrepreneur Association's (FEAI) mission is to inspire and empower women from around the world to build successful businesses. FEAI provides weekly videos, an online community, master classes, a monthly magazine, and a variety of social media to help inspire women to succeed in business.

Women Entrepreneurs of America, Inc. (www.weainc.webs.com): Women Entrepreneurs of America, Inc. was established in November 2002 by Yolanda Lamar-Wilder. This organization guides and supports women in the pursuit of business success, offering workshops, seminars, and consulting services. Monthly business luncheons and forums, self-promotion, and networking opportunities are available and encouraged.

The National Association of Negro Business And Professional Women's Clubs, Inc. (www.nanbpwc.org): NANBPWC, Inc. was founded in 1935 to promote and protect the interests of business and professional women, to serve as advisors for young people seeking to enter business and the professions, to improve the quality of life in our local and global communities, and to foster good fellowship.

Young Female Entrepreneurs (www.youngfemaleentrepreneurs. com): YFE is an online network connecting entrepreneurial women in their 20s and 30s with new people, brands, and headlines that help them start and grow businesses.

Online Professional Networking Sites

In addition to connecting with and learning from business organizations, private practice lactation consultants will want to be active in profession-related online support groups. Here are some options:

LACTNET (community.lsoft.com/SCRIPTS/WA-LSOFTDONATIONS. EXE?A0=lactnet): Lactnet is a LISTSERV® email list for anyone involved in providing support to mothers in breastfeeding their infants and young children. Lactnet's members include lactation consultants, lay breastfeeding counselors, nurses, doctors, midwives, public health advocates, pharmacologists, marketing experts, writers, journalists, scientists, dieticians, and doulas. The list, which has been operating for almost 20 years, has over 4,200 subscribers from countries covering every continent except Antarctica. The type of discussions that occur on the Lactnet list include brainstorming difficult breastfeeding problems with the client's permission to post; debating ethical issues; sharing information on newly published articles, books, or research; dialogue about controversial issues; networking; and sharing emotional and informational support among members. In addition to daily postings and digests, Lactnet has public list archives that provide members, as well as the general public, with a wealth of information and inspiration. Lactnet was founded in 1995 by Kathleen Bruce, a Vermont nurse and International Board Certified Lactation Consultant (IBCLC), and Kathleen Auerbach, PhD, IBCLC, who wanted to create a network of support for isolated lactation consultants who lacked the benefit of local peers. To subscribe, send mail to LISTSERV@ COMMUNITY.LSOFT.COM with the command (subscribe) in the e-mail message body.

LCinPP (www.lcinpp.com): This group is for participants of the annual Lactation Consultant in Private Practice Workshops to encourage, inform, and support one another. The Lactation Consultant in Private Practice workshops are an absolute must for those looking into or already established in private practice. Terriann Shell writes, "Many lactation consultants are excellent at helping mothers overcome breastfeeding challenges, but lack business management skills to be in private practice. This is the concept behind the Lactation Consultant in Private Practice workshop that has been held annually since 1987. Started by Kay Hoover and Chris Mulford, the workshop features business-building skills, along with networking, where wanna-bes, newbies, and pros learn from each other's experiences. Lactation consultants explore how new and changing technology and social media can be used for more efficient home visiting or office consultations. Lactation sessions focus on areas not covered in typical breastfeeding conferences, like challenges that arise after mothers leave the birthing facility. Consultants discuss the resolution of the ethical dilemmas unique to private practice. The sisterhood of private practice is continued throughout the year on Yahoo and Facebook groups that are open only to previous attendees" (personal communication, Jan. 15, 2014). The LCinPP Workshops are held in February or March of each year in Philadelphia, PA.

PP IBCLC (www.facebook.com/groups/232881560127082/): This is a closed group on Facebook for IBCLCs in private practice.

Breastfeeding Network–IBCLC in PP (www.facebook.com/ groups/545691455480002/): Another closed group on Facebook for IBCLCs in private practice.

Paperless IBCLC (www.facebook.com/groups/238456043009308/): A closed Facebook group for IBCLCs that are looking for an alternative method of keeping private practice files in order. Please message Sarah Eichler with your name as it appears on the IBCLE registry, if it is different than your Facebook name.

IBCLC in WIC (www.facebook.com/groups/279719815484019/): This is a closed Facebook group for IBCLCs working with the Women, Infants, and Children's Program.

Breastfeeding Educators and Lactation Consultants Unite (www. facebook.com/groups/bfeducatorsunite/): A closed Facebook group for breastfeeding educators and lactation consultants for support, encouragement, and resources. You must be credentialed in some way as a breastfeeding educator (RN, LVN, CBE, CLC, LLL etc.) or IBCLC to join the group. If you do not have your credentials on your Facebook bio, please send your name and credentials to admin@askthelactationconsultant.com upon asking to join the group.

Breastfeeding Network—Lactation Support Professionals (www. facebook.com/groups/206576862839048/): This is a closed Facebook group to allow lactation professionals to assist mothers and babies, learn from one another, and grow in professional education.

HBLC'S (groups.yahoo.com/neo/groups/HBLCs/info): Started in 2000, this is a closed list only for Lactation Consultants who currently practice in hospitals.

Babyconferences (groups.yahoo.com/neo/groups/BabyConferencesinfo): Begun in 1999, this email list is for those who wish to be notified of professional conferences relating to the fields of lactation and maternal and newborn nursing. Members can post about any and all upcoming conferences.

IBCLC-PP (groups.yahoo.com/neo/groups/IBCLC-PP/info): A discussion group started in 2002 for private practice IBCLCs and those who intend to enter private practice in the immediate future.

LACTPSYCH (groups.yahoo.com/neo/groups/LactPsych/info): LactPsych is an international email discussion group for professionals working in the field of lactational psychology. It was founded on May 23, 2005, by Cynthia Good Mojab, MS, IBCLC, RLC, CATSM, who continues to serve as its moderator. The purposes of LactPsych include discussion of topics within and related to lactational psychology, networking, peer support, and discussion of concerns and ideas for developing, expanding, and improving the multidisciplinary work done by dual professionals in the field of lactational psychology. Members have dual credentials, work experience, and/or education in the fields of psychology and breastfeeding. Most, but not all, members of LactPsych are International Board Certified Lactation Consultants. Professionals interested in becoming members of LactPsych may send an email to Cynthia Good Mojab at lactpsych-owner@yahoogroups.com describing their credentials, experience, and education in both fields to determine if they and LactPsych are a good match. Membership in LactPsych is currently restricted to professionals with substantial interest, credentials, experience, and education in lactational psychology.

Professional Organizations

Lactation consultants are a part of the healthcare team, and as such, have their own professional organizations. Membership and active participation in these organizations should be considered, as it is the grass-roots consultant that helps to change policy, laws, practices, and other areas in which these organizations are actively working.

International Lactation Consultant Association (www.ilca.org): The International Lactation Consultant Association (ILCA) is the professional association for International Board Certified Lactation Consultants and other healthcare professionals who care for breastfeeding families. ILCA membership is open to all who support and promote breastfeeding; you do not need to be an IBCLC to become a member. ILCA keeps members informed of the latest happenings in the field of lactation consulting through the *Journal of Human Lactation*. Members receive a free listing in "Find a Lactation Consultant" online referral directory (only for IBCLCs); "Worksite Lactation Support Directory" online referral for employers (only for IBCLCs); and "Clinical Instruction Directory" (IBCLCs qualified to supervise aspiring lactation consultants who are acquiring clinical experience); an e-newsletter, *ILCAlert*; discussion boards; Listserv message alerts; website announcements; annual and regional conferences (with discounts for ILCA members); Worldwide Education Calendar; online Continuing Education for instant CERP credit (discounted for ILCA members); and online bookstore with exam prep materials for ILCA members, business materials, ILCA publications, WBW and IBCLC Day items, and much more (with discounts for members).

United States Lactation Consultant Association (www.uslca.org): The United States Lactation Consultant Association (USLCA) was the first national affiliate of ILCA. In July 2014, USLCA announced their intention to be a freestanding organization in the United States. As a member of USLCA, you receive benefits such as subscription to the peer-reviewed *Journal of Clinical Lactation*, including both hard copy and online access; *eNews*, USLCA's monthly newsletter; discounts on online and recorded webinars with the opportunity to earn CERPs; press releases on current issues of importance to IBCLCs; information on pursuing licensure and insurance reimbursement; and representation in U.S. governmental and professional organizations to advocate for the IBCLC to be the gold standard of lactation professionals.

Professional Resources

Many lactation consultants in general and private practice LCs in particular have extensive (and expensive) library resources within their office. Keeping current can prove to be a challenge for many. Online access to basic resources is valuable to those LCs not in their office or who are somehow caught without the latest research-based information. Here are a few valuable resources:

LACTMED (toxnet.nlm.nih.gov/cgi-bin/sis/htmlgen?LACT): LactMed, a free online database with information on drugs and lactation, is one of the newest additions to the National Library of Medicine's TOXNET system, a Web-based collection of resources covering toxicology, chemical safety, and environmental health. Geared to the healthcare practitioner and nursing mother, LactMed contains multiple drug records and is updated monthly. It includes information on maternal drug levels in breast milk, levels in infant blood, potential effects in breastfeeding infants and on lactation itself, the American Academy of Pediatrics category indicating the level of compatibility of the drug with breastfeeding, and alternate drugs to consider. References are included, as is nomenclature information, such as the drug's Chemical Abstract Service's (CAS) Registry number and its broad drug class. Free apps for iPhones and Androids are available.

InfantRisk Center (www.infantrisk.com): The InfantRisk Center at Texas Tech University Health Sciences Center, Lubbock, TX, USA, is a call center (806-352-2519) based solely on evidence-based medicine and research. Thomas W. Hale, RPh, PhD, Professor of Pediatrics at Texas Tech University School of Medicine, is the Executive Director of the InfantRisk Center. The InfantRisk Center is dedicated to providing current and accurate information to pregnant and breastfeeding mothers and healthcare professionals. It serves as a training center for medical and pharmacy students and medical residents in the use of drugs in pregnant and breastfeeding mothers. It has recently started an extensive program in clinical research, with several large clinical trials completed last year, and several more to begin soon. The InfantRisk Helpline answers questions about the use of medications during pregnancy and breastfeeding, nausea and vomiting during pregnancy, and alcohol, substance abuse, and depression during pregnancy and breastfeeding.

Webforum At Infantrisk Center (www.infantrisk.com/content/ webforum): The web forum consists of two sections, one is the standard drug section where only healthcare professionals are permitted to ask questions, but all can review the questions and responses. Lactation consultants, LLL Leaders, physicians, pharmacists, nurses, and other professionals in this field may post a question, particularly if it is something new or not well covered in the three books by Dr. Hale.

Local and State Coalitions

In addition to the international and national breastfeeding coalition support organizations (Appendix A), lactation consultants will want to consider state, area, and local coalitions that support, protect, and promote breastfeeding. Doing so promotes networking with those like-minded professions in your locale. It also promotes your visibility in the area and can be used in press releases, blogs, or newsletter updates to show community dedication and volunteerism. A listing of these different organizations can be found in the Appendix B.

Experienced LCs Share

From whom do you seek your professional peer support?

The lactation consultants represented here seem to have found a wide variety of support to learn from, receive feedback from, and gather and share information with.

Other IBCLCs were frequently listed as a source of support, although these were not usually in the same vicinity as the private practice LC.

Coalitions and taskforces in the area provided support for some.

Online support was the most frequently mentioned, with Facebook and Yahoo groups for lactation issues and for private practice discussed.

Many of the IBCLCs have attended the Lactation Consultant in Private Practice (LCinPP) workshops and find a great support system through both the annual on-site sharing and the daily online Yahoo group for attendees.

ILCA was said to provide support in the form of conferences, webinars, and discussion groups.

Lactnet was listed as not only a source of support, but as an educational venue.

Many named specific IBCLCs with advanced practice as their mentors and supporters.

One IBCLC mentioned Women In Business and Women's Chamber of Commerce in her community as a good source of support and education. Although members of these groups do not have the lactation background, there is a great deal of commonality as business owners and sole practitioners.

Private Practice Self-Check

Are you a member of a professional business organization for women? If not, which one(s) will you join?

Are you a member of an Internet group for lactation professionals? If not, which Internet group(s) will you join?

Are you a member of a lactation professional association? If not, which one(s) will you join?

Are you a member of a state or local breastfeeding task force? If not, which one(s) will you join?

In what other ways can you obtain valuable information on running a business, networking with peers, and keeping up to date on new information in your field?

Chapter Ten. My Internet Presence

No man is an island entire of itself; every man is a piece of the continent, a part of the main.

~John Donne

The 2013 figures for Internet presence and social media are astounding. If your private practice does not have an Internet presence yet, take a look at some of the reasons you need one:

- Internet—2.7 billion people use the Internet worldwide. Of those, 191 million are U.S. based, 73% use social networking sites, and 73% connect online at least once per day. On social media, 98% of 18-24 year olds are active regularly in one platform or another.

- YouTube—One billion users worldwide; four billion videos viewed daily; 92 billion pages viewed each month.

- Instagram—150 million members sharing 55 million photos and videos each day. Every second, 8000 users "like" a photo.

- LinkedIn—260 million subscribers, 173 new members each day (that's eight per minute). More than 42% of users update their profile regularly.

- Twitter—750 million subscribers, sending 500 million tweets per day. The fastest growing age demographic is the 55-64 year olds. Average number of tweets per account is 208, and 34% of marketers are targeting Twitter to generate leads.

- Pinterest—20 million subscribers, 80% are women.

- Facebook—1.23 billion users, 169 million are U.S. based. This is 11% of the population of the Earth! Average number of friends per user is almost 200. 751 million are mobile users. 23% check their account more than five times per day. 74% of marketers believe Facebook is important for their marketing strategy.

- Vine—40 million members share videos worldwide.

- Snapchat—4.6 million members share 350 million photos each day.

- Google+—One billion users, 67% are male, 56% are 45-54 year olds. Predicted to surpass Facebook by 2016. 40% of marketers use this platform.

- Wikipedia—Over 476 million unique visitors per month visit the 17 million articles on this site.

- Flickr—Over 3,000 pictures uploaded to site per minute, over five billion photos are on the site.

- Up-and-coming sites: StumbleUpon, Delicious, GoogleReader, GoogleBookmarks, Blinklist, Posterous, Tumblr, Sphinn, MSNReporter, HackerNews, Reddit, Digg, MySpace, Slideshare.

- The top ten most engaged countries for social networking include Israel, Argentina, Russia, Turkey, Chile, The Philippines, Colombia, Peru, Venezuela, Canada, and the United States (Ajmera, 2014; Bullas, 2014; Harden, 2014).

To put these figures in perspective, as of 2012 the world population was over seven billion. That means Facebook has one-sixth of the world population as members; Google+ and YouTube have one-seventh each, and one-ninth of the world population sends tweets on Twitter! This is especially staggering when you consider that 1.5 billion people in the world live without electricity or technology; that is approximately one-fourth of the world's population!

The Generational Differences

There is a tremendous amount of research available on the differences in the generations. Here is the categorization of ages at this time:

- G.I. Generation: Born 1901–1924, current ages 90 and older

- Silent Generation: Born 1925–1942, current ages 89–72

- Baby Boomer Generation: Born 1943–1964, current ages 50–71

- Generation X: Born 1965–1979, current ages 35–49

- Generation Y or Millennial Generation: Born 1980-2000, current ages 14-34

According to the Centers for Disease Control and Prevention (DHHS, 2012), there are about 83 million mothers in the U.S. today. Millennial mothers are the largest percentage of this population, with 32.5 million. Generation X mothers account for another 22 million. These are the two primary generational groups that lactation consultants work with regularly. The grandmothers of the new babies fall into the Boomer Generation and occasionally the Silent Generation.

The Silent Generation were the youngest parents in U.S. history. They were the children of the Great Depression and World War II. This hardworking generation birthed the Baby Boomers.

Baby Boomers wanted to have and be better than their parents. Commonly called the "me generation," Boomers identified strongly with what they did at work, valuing long work hours and upward mobility. This generation was known for rebelling against the constraints of their parents.

Generation X children grew up during the Boomer consciousness revolution, when the welfare of children was not a top priority. Many were latchkey children since childcare was not widely available. Many Gen Xers learned to distrust institutions and the family. Many Xers dated later and married later. The families of this generation were the first to experience geographic dispersion, without their extended family in the same town. Involvement with their children grew during this age.

Millennials arrived at a time when parents wanted hands-on parenting. Babies were special and child abuse and safety became hot topics, as well as the teaching of virtues and values to their children. Millennials tend to have a very strong, close relationship with their parents and family members. Due to the protective parenting of the Gen Xers, Millennials tend to have a sense of entitlement. More than half of the Millennial generation were raised by a single parent. Fifty-three percent of Millennial mothers are single. Being a good parent is one of the highest priorities for these mothers.

Digital Motherhood

The Gen Xers and Millennial mothers seek healthcare information and assistance on the Internet, before turning to any other source. Over 90% follow what other mothers recommend to them online. Mothers seeking assistance with breastfeeding online desire several things: (1) humor, done right; (2) simplicity, offering several solutions to the problem they are researching; and (3) sincerity and credibility, regardless of the topic (Fleschner, 2008; Oblinger, 2003; Strauss, 2005). Most moms go online several times each day for social networking, blogs, and to research information. They put a great deal of time and effort into choosing the best for themselves and their families, and they want a say in the decision and outcome. TV has taken a backseat to learning online. These two generations have never been without technology in the form of computers, the Internet, and social media. Multitasking is a way of life. These mothers can listen to music, send instant messages, breastfeed their baby, and chat on the phone–all at the same time! It may be disconcerting to the Boomer-age lactation consultant, or even considered rude, when noting these behaviors during a consultation. Typing is preferred to handwriting, since keyboard learning occurred from preschool (or younger) and penmanship has never been stressed. Almost constant technological connection is required by the Gen X and Millennial mothers, as they desire information when they need it, using smart phones, texting, instant messaging, laptops, tablets, and real-time discussions like Skype or FaceTime. With this expectation, there is little tolerance for delays. They desire 24/7 services and quick responses.

Delays cause dissatisfaction and disengagement. And word of mouth travels online very quickly (Fleschner, 2008; Oblinger, 2003; Strauss, 2005).

For younger, first-time mothers, the Internet is often the primary source of information (Bernhardt & Felter, 2004). Because more than half of these mothers return to paid employment, they spend less time networking with other mothers of young children. The need for increased informal support, advice, and interaction with other mothers has driven the Gen X and Millennial mothers online to seek this support. Drentea and Moren-Cross (2005) found that the Internet allows geographically diverse mothers to come together and create a community of caring and information sharing. In a 1999 study, Bailey found that the Internet was effective "in providing new mothers access to alternative information sources, which increased their real sense of empowerment and helped to ameliorate some of the potentially alienating aspects of life as a new mother."

Although social media via the Internet allows new mothers to connect with their own mothers and grandmothers more frequently, these same mothers seek more up-to-date mothering and parenting information online. The information shared by close family is felt to be out-of-date (O'Connor & Madge, 2004). Today's new mothers are no longer satisfied with a book or magazine description of parenting, but require more experience-based information. They want to connect with others in similar situations. In their review of literature on parents use of the Internet, Plantin and Daneback (2009) describe the demographic profile of the average Internet-using parent as a young (under age 35), white, middle-class woman who uses the web to search for health information and to visit parenting web sites. The researchers felt this confirmed the mother's offline behavior for taking on the main responsibility for hands-on care of the family. The sheer variety of conversational topics discussed in forums amazed the researchers, prompting them to state, "it is difficult to imagine any single community service providing, in such a timely manner, the diverse amount of information and support that these women exchange on a daily basis" (Dunham et al., 1998).

The Internet has been perceived as a quick way to access health and parenting information, confirming the information provided by a primary care provider or seeking alternative treatments and suggestions. Mothers value the ability to cross-check information between various websites. Because there is a sense of confidentiality on the Internet, mothers can search for information on sensitive or embarrassing topics. As lactation professionals, we are concerned about the quality of breastfeeding information provided on the many websites available to new mothers. However, at least three-fourths of the population thinks the Internet is a reliable and credible source of information.

There are consumer-based tools that have been developed to assess the credibility of the information on the websites, such as DISCERN, NetScoring, and MedCertain. However, few consumers know of and utilize the criteria presented with these tools. Shaikh and Scott (2005) performed an analysis of breastfeeding websites for accuracy. Of the 40 websites most frequently accessed by mothers, they found the majority of the website content provided was accurate information and complied with the International Code of Marketing of Breast-Milk Substitutes. However, compliance with the Health on the Net Code of Conduct (HONcode) was far less. The HONcode is a rating instrument specific to healthcare-related websites, created in 1996 by the Geneva-based Health on the Net Foundation. It contains guidelines to rate sites, including:

- **Authority:** Does the site describe the qualifications of the authors?

- **Complementarity:** Does the information support, not replace, the doctor-patient relationship?

- **Privacy:** Does the site respect the privacy and confidentiality of personal data submitted to the site by the visitor?

- **Attribution:** Does the site cite the source(s) of published information and date medical and health pages?

- **Justifiability:** Does the site back up claims relating to benefits and performance?

- **Transparency:** Does the site indicate who created the site and give accurate and complete contact information?

- **Financial disclosure:** Does the site identify funding sources?

- **Advertising policy:** Does the site clearly distinguish advertising from editorial content?

Lactation Online

The Internet has the ability to reach large numbers of new mothers at a relatively low cost for both providers and consumers. Pate (2009) demonstrated that Internet-based interventions may be an appealing option as compared to provider-based breastfeeding education and support. There are, at this time, a shortage of studies conducted based on rigorous design and comprehensive analysis to show that Internet breastfeeding interventions make a difference in the general population.

Regardless, mothers seek breastfeeding information via the Internet; experience worldwide demonstrates this. And it has been available since the mid1990's, starting first with Parent-L, Lactnet, and BFAR (breastfeeding after reduction) (Audelo, 2014). Lactation consultants need to be savvy to the Internet and the sources of breastfeeding support available to today's mothers. Former U.S. Surgeon General Dr. Regina Benjamin, in her 2011 Call to Action, stated that social media was an important tool for reaching breastfeeding mothers (McCann & McCulloch, 2012).

In a 2012 article in *Breastfeeding Medicine,* Dr. Todd Wolynn emphasized the new information paradigm of PUSH vs. PULL. In the old information paradigm, information was sought from the library, written publications, and books. Then came the ability to Google it online and "pull" that information from an Internet source. The new paradigm "pushes" information to seekers through newsfeeds in Facebook and Twitter posts. Wolynn states, "We have to go where the people are, make ourselves available and relevant and valuable in their social networks and in their social media platforms, and then push our information to them every month, every week, every day. We have to show up in their Facebook feeds between their friends, their family members, their co-workers, and their favorite bands, as a constant presence, and so as a trusted source, in their digital lives." This is so very vital and pertinent to the lactation consultants trying to reach new mothers today.

Being Professional

The American Medical Association has developed an Opinion Paper on *Professionalism in the Use of Social Media* (2010). You can easily substitute "lactation consultant" for "physician" throughout this opinion. It suggests several considerations when maintaining an online presence:

- Physicians should be cognizant of **standards of patient privacy and confidentiality** that must be maintained in all environments, including online, and must refrain from posting identifiable patient information online.

- When using the Internet for social networking, physicians should use **privacy settings to safeguard personal information** and content to the extent possible, but should realize that privacy settings are not absolute and that once on the Internet, content is likely to be there permanently. Thus, physicians should **routinely monitor** their own Internet presence to ensure that the personal and professional information on their own sites, and to the extent possible, content posted about them by others, is accurate and appropriate.

- If they interact with patients on the Internet, physicians must **maintain appropriate boundaries of the patient-physician relationship** in accordance with professional ethical guidelines, just as they would in any other context.

- To maintain appropriate professional boundaries, physicians should **consider separating personal and professional content online.**

- When physicians see content posted by colleagues that appears **unprofessional,** they have a **responsibility to bring**

that content to the attention of the individual, so that he/she can remove it and/or take other appropriate actions. If the behavior significantly violates professional norms and the individual does not take appropriate action to resolve the situation, the physician should report the matter to appropriate authorities.

- Physicians must recognize that **actions online and content posted may negatively affect their reputations** among patients and colleagues, may have consequences for their medical careers (particularly for physicians-in-training and medical students), and can undermine public trust in the medical profession.

Be sure to read the *Code of Professional Conduct, Scope of Practice, and Standards of Practice for IBCLCs* in order to apply them to your online presence. Although these documents do not discuss online and social media presence as such, they do provide the guidelines for practice, ethics, and care that IBCLCs are to uphold.

Robyn Kaplan, CLE, IBCLC, in a 2012 post to LactationMatters, listed several ways to use social media effectively as a lactation consultant:

- Create a social media plan appropriate to your specific practice and the time you have available to spend online.

- Decide who your target audience is and the purpose of your engagement.

- Choose one or two social media platforms that you feel are manageable and plan for the amount of time you want to dedicate to social media each week.

- Go to those platforms and spend time just watching and listening, which allows you to define what your audience is seeking.

- Keep in mind that social media is all about sharing information. While you don't want to give away everything you know, the more information you benevolently share online, the more appreciative your audience will be and the more they will engage your platform in the future.

In the Nursing profession, there are cases where Registered Nurses have been issued warnings, legal consequences, and loss of practice privileges to certain locations when confidentiality has been breached online. In one case described by Spector and Kappel (2012), a nursing student wanted to remember the three-year-old patient she had been caring for, who was receiving chemotherapy for leukemia at a local hospital. When taking his photograph, the room number was visible in the background. The photo was then posted on Facebook for friends to see, with the student commenting about how brave her patient was and how proud she was to be a nursing student. Like many users of Facebook and other social media, she did not know that others can access posts even when appropriate privacy settings are in place. In this case, someone forwarded the information to a nurse at that hospital, who then contacted her supervisor. Since the nursing school had clear policies about not breaching confidentiality and HIPAA violations, the student was expelled from the program. The nursing program was no longer allowed to provide clinicals at that hospital.

Several state Boards of Nursing report complaints against nurses related to social media, placing them in the following categories (Spector & Kappel, 2012). Again, substitute lactation consultant for nurse here, as good guidance in your social media dealings.

- **Breach of privacy or confidentiality against patients.** Any patient information gained during the course of care must be safeguarded by the nurse, and confidential information can only be shared with informed consent. Federal law reinforces confidentiality and privacy through HIPAA.

- **Failure to report others' violations of privacy against patients.** It is imperative for nurses to report any violation of patient privacy or confidentiality from others.

- **Lateral violence against colleagues.** Online posts about co-workers, even if posted from home during non-work hours, may constitute lateral violence. Lateral violence includes the disruptive behaviors of intimidation and bullying, as well as slander and libel.

- **Communication against employers.** There is a fine line between free speech and complaining about an employer on social media. The courts are deciding cases such as these at this very time.

- **Boundary violations.** Online contact with patients or former patients blurs the distinction between a professional and personal relationship. These professional boundaries are the spaces between the nurse's power and the patient's vulnerability.

- **Employer/faculty use of social media against employees/ students.** Legislation was introduced or considered in at least 36 states in 2013 to prevent employers from demanding new employee passwords to social media sites. Ten states– Arkansas, Colorado, Illinois, Nevada, New Jersey, New Mexico, Oregon, Utah, Vermont and Washington–enacted legislation in 2013. Legislation has been introduced or is pending in at least 28 states, and enacted in Louisiana, Maine (authorizes study), Oklahoma, Tennessee, and Wisconsin in 2014. For the latest information on your state, go to http://www.ncsl.org

McCann and McCulloch (2012) remind lactation consultants that "because social media interactions do not permit a comprehensive intake, history, and assessment, IBCLCs are advised to not offer direct clinical advice to a mother in a social media venue…which should be educational and supportive in nature."

Videoconferencing

Videoconferencing may involve the electronic exchange of health information protected under the U.S. HIPAA law. If you use videoconferencing, take security measures to ensure unauthorized parties cannot record or listen in on a session, storing and identifying each session in a secure and proper manner, and having a procedure for initiating and receiving video calls. Consider also security features for text chat, screen sharing, and file transfers. HIPAA's Security Rule does not require encryption if you can prove it is not reasonable or appropriate to do so. However, it is a very good idea to encrypt data whenever possible; doing so exempts HIPAA-covered entities from the Breach Rule if a data breach occurs. There are many services available to you if you are providing online consultations through videoconferencing. Check out securevideo.com, lifesize.com, imeet.com, verizonbusiness.com, brothercloud.com, avispl.com, or vsee.com.

It is important to know that smart phones are not usually encrypted and are not secure for sharing HIPAA covered information. In fact, "most mobile phones on the market today meet no more than 40% of security requirements–such as those called for by HIPPA…in the out-of-the-box configurations. And even after being manually configured, only iPhone and BlackBerry smartphones typically achieve about 60% of standards," according to Neil Versel (2012). Think you don't have HIPAA-compliant private health information (PHI) on your phone? Think again…if you have clients email you with test results, pictures of their breastfeeding issues, or their address, telephone number, credit card number, or any other private information. Your smartphone will also contain that information if you use some form of syncing your email to your phone. So if you lose your phone, it is stolen, or the information is breached, you have a data breach and HIPAA violation. Art Gross states, "Without having a startup password and encryption on the phone, you are looking at having to send a breach notification to each one of your patients…and tens of thousands of dollars in forensics to determine which patients need to be notified…and possibly offering credit monitoring services" (2011). The HIPAA Security Rule outlines standards designed to protect electronic PHI and states, "Unauthorized disclosure of PHI is a risk because mobile devices store data on the device itself in one of two way: (1) within the computer onboard memory or (2) within the SIM card or memory chip," reports Catherine Barrett of the American Bar Association (2011). Barrett goes on to describe clinicians who are "far more likely to use their own personal mobile devices, rather than employer-issued mobile devices, to access and exchange ePHI, with an estimated 81% using personal mobile devices" (2011).

How can private practice LCs prevent a data breach of ePHI? Barrett describes using technical safeguards, such as encryption, installation and regular updates of anti-malicious software (malware) on mobile devices, installing firewalls, having backup capabilities, such as off-site data and/ or private clouds, and use of secure encrypted Hypertext Transfer Protocol Secure (HTTPS) similar to those used in banking and financial transactions (2011). A full description of the HIPAA security requirements for ePHI can be found on the Department of Health and Human Services website (2006).

The November 2012 issue of the *Journal of Human Lactation* dealt with online breastfeeding support issues. Four articles in this issue provided excellent information specific to telehealth, videoconferencing, and breastfeeding. Here is a quick recap of each article:

Macnab, Rojjanasrirat, and Sanders (2012) described their experiences using real-time videoconferencing for lactation consultations. They shared that the vast majority of mothers are open to this type of conferencing via the Internet, and most are pleased with the results following the consult. Problems they experienced with videoconferencing include poor pictures and sound, Internet variability, and the inability to perform the physical assessments lactation consultants might be used to, i.e., suck assessments.

Ahmed and Ouzzani (2012) tested the feasibility of web-based monitoring among breastfeeding mothers to examine the feasibility, usability, and acceptability of this method, termed LACTOR, based on a breastfeeding diary. Results showed that most mothers felt they did not need to learn many breastfeeding skills prior to the use of LACTOR, but that the monitoring was beneficial in assisting to track infant feeding patterns and detect breastfeeding problems early.

Rojjanasrirat, Nelson, and Wambach (2012) used four real-time videoconferencing sessions to deliver lactation support to ten mothers in their own homes. Breastfeeding problems, such as latch, suck problems, jaundice, and cracked or sore nipples, were easily identified by the telehealth IBCLC. Input from the mothers after the sessions revealed that "mothers were particularly enthusiastic about not having to travel with their young infant to receive help," and they were comfortable discussing breastfeeding concerns via the Internet.

In an excellent article by McCann & McCulloch (2012), they encouraged lactation professionals to learn to use web-based methods to engage the breastfeeding community online. "Regardless of the chosen platform, social media is most successful when it promotes engagement with a target audience." Facebook, Twitter, Pinterest, and blogs were identified "as useful platforms for connecting to breastfeeding mothers."

Blogging

Is blogging right for you? Consider these questions before you answer that question. Do you enjoy writing…a lot of writing? What is your message, what do you want to communicate to your audience? Do you have great communication skills? Are you a better writer than speaker? Do you want to be the central voice on your website? Do you have the motivation to begin and continue to run a blog? Do you have lots of time to devote to blogging? Are you able to take negative comments and critiques? Are you willing to consistently be in the public spotlight? Do you possess technical skills to work with web-based software? Do you have a sense of humor to apply to the blog? Are you willing to learn? Do you enjoy reading the blogs of others? Are you an organized, creative, and social person? Are you willing to be honest and transparent?

Blogs are time-consuming to keep up with and can take months (or longer) to "take off" in the public view. They may not be suitable for every practitioner. You might need to assess your needs, personality, creativity, and desire to share before beginning a blog.

Generally, blog posts contain less than 600 words and are written in a conversational tone. Geared toward your target audience, blog posts should provide value to your website visitors, familiarize them with your services and your professional viewpoint, and build your practice. Be sure to read, share, and comment on other breastfeeding blogs. Use Twitter to announce your blog, pin it to a Pinterest board, link to it in a Facebook newsfeed, and spread the word through other platforms of social media.

Email

Email is a mainstay of communication nowadays. Many people no longer write letters by hand, even thank you notes, but prefer to email their thoughts and thanks. Michael Hyatt (2007) provides excellent etiquette suggestions for email. The following lactation consultant suggestions are adapted from Hyatt's work:

- "To" vs "CC." The names included in the "To" field of an email should be those whom you expect to read and respond. Only "CC" those people you want to keep in the loop.

- Keep your email messages brief and to the point. The communication should be clear, expected actions or responses identified, and the email should address a single subject. A long, complex email is easily set aside until a "better time" to deal with it.

- Remember that our new mothers expect timely responses. Don't wait a day or two to respond to their emails.

- Use your spellcheck religiously. Misspelled and grammatically incorrect words give a very unprofessional look to your work.

- Don't write in all caps–this is considered the digital equivalent of yelling.

- Watch your tone. Remember that your recipient cannot see your face and body language or hear your vocal inflections. Avoid sarcasm.

- Avoid replying in criticism or anger. This is not professional, can cause the loss of clients, and can create a negative reputation that lasts a long time.

- Use your professional credentials to create a signature line, complete with the appropriate contact information.

- Re-read your email before hitting the send button. You think faster than you can type and words can be left out, used in the wrong form, or misspelled.

Hashtags

What began as a way to search posts on Twitter, hashtags (# sign before a series of letters) now allow a global search for any social post. Include hashtags in all your posts. To create a new hashtag, avoid using spaces. Even if your hashtag contains multiple words, group them all together. If you want to differentiate between words, use capitals instead (#BreastfeedingPerspectives). Uppercase letters will not alter your search results. Numbers are supported, so tweet about #50reasonstobreastfeed to your heart's content. However, punctuation marks are not, so commas, periods, exclamation points, question marks, and apostrophes are out. Forget about asterisks, ampersands, or any other special characters. Keep in mind that the @ symbol does something completely different. Using @ before a person's Twitter handle will tweet her directly, letting her know you have written to her via the @Connect tab. A hashtag will not. There is no preset list of hashtags. Create a brand new hashtag simply by putting the hash before a series of words, and if it hasn't been used before, you've invented your own hashtag.

Facebook

If you're looking for a general overview of how to use Facebook to help your business grow, the fundamentals can be found at www.facebook.com/business/overview. The step-by-step directions on setting up a business page are user-friendly. You can request a web address to match your practice's name. Facebook will help you build your target audience, share your page and invite business contacts. Advice is given on creating compelling content for your page, advertising if you desire and building your own ads. Tools for measuring your effectiveness and reach are included in the package.

When initially setting up your page, you will choose the category of your business from a drop-down menu and name your page. You will add profile and cover photos and basic information about your practice. You can always add more about your practice later. "Like" your own page, then send it out into the social media atmosphere!

It isn't the number of "likes" your page receives that is important; it's all about interactions. For Facebook, weekends and late afternoon or evening are the times when page administrators are least likely to add a new post, even though those are the highest interaction times. Thursdays have the highest number of posts, but the lowest interaction rate. To generate more interaction, use photos to evoke emotion and grab attention. Facebook status updates (or posts) allow users to discuss online their thoughts, whereabouts, new business offerings, or other important information. It is usually short and informative, without going into great detail. However, it has been shown by Facebook that longer status updates create more interaction, longer than your typical 140-character limitation for Twitter posts.

One of the social media predictions for the next several years is that you will have to pay for a Facebook site. The availability of free accounts will still exist, but to get your posts seen by potential new clients, expect to pay for it.

Google+

This new search engine's attempt to create a social network that rivals Facebook is quickly growing. Launched in June of 2011, it has grown to over 1 billion users. Google+ shows higher engagement than other social media platforms and is beginning to integrate other cloud products like documents, calendar, and reader. You can disable reshares of your post, use "circles" for following others, and have a set of hotkey shortcuts. Understanding "circles" is essential to mastering Google+. Circles allow users to drag-and-drop their friends into different friend groups, such as family, business, friends, or whatever category you create. These circles give you more control over who sees what portion of your site content, as well as what content pops up in your stream (newslead). The search feature delves through people, pages, and content, and searches can be saved for easy retrieval.

The Google+ Hangouts is a novel twist on the traditional video group chat, although if you have never used the Google Talk feature, you will need to install a small piece of software before Hangouts will work. The newest features to be added to Hangouts include integration with Google Docs, the ability to screen share, and a sketchpad feature.

Picassa, owned by Google, provides the power technology for the fully built photo album available in Google+. You can upload photos and create albums, as well as edit those photos within the application.

Using the "profile and privacy" tab located in the Google+ settings page, you can edit the visibility of every part of your profile, manage your circles, change your network visibility, adjust your photo settings, and review those settings as someone else would see them.

In order to be ranked on Google searches, Google+ must be a part of your social media sites; their posts count towards your search ranking.

Instagram

Instagram, first launched in October 2010, is a free online photo and video sharing and social networking service. It uses a cell phone camera to take pictures. Users can apply photo filters and share the pictures on the web to Twitter, Facebook, Tumblr, and Flickr. A distinctive feature is that photos are square instead of the 4:3 aspect ratio typically used by mobile device cameras. Users are also able to record and share short videos lasting up to 15 seconds. Hashtags are used in this forum to connect those with similar interests. The application is compatible with iPhone, iPad, or iPod Touch and Android devices.

Because social networks are becoming much more image-driven, Instagram is a popular business site. You can create an account name, add a profile photo, create a short text description of your practice, and include several hashtags. There are a variety of photo image tools to ramp up your photos. The site includes tagging, liking, commenting, and more. Getting started is easy; just follow the step-by-step directions at the site. The first step says, "Consider how Instagram fits into your overall brand marketing strategy. Is your objective to increase awareness, shift perception, or reach a new audience? Pick a goal or two that can be achieved by connecting with Instagram's highly visual and creative community" (www.instagram.com/gettingstarted).

LinkedIn

LinkedIn is a professional social networking site, allowing you to showcase your practice and connect with your target audience. Business pages are easy to create and raise brand awareness, promote career opportunities, and educate potential customers about your products and services. The more followers you have, the easier it becomes to get viral reach and engagement. You can generate business leads and strengthen current customer relationships by sharing valuable content via company updates.

You can create a free business page with a company profile. Then add a banner, logo, and links to your other marketing channels, such as email, newsletters, blogs, and your website. Daily postings update your followers with news of the practice, breastfeeding articles, or by asking followers to comment on questions or topics. You can include images, infographics, videos, slideshows, and presentations. And you can track engagement on posts, followers, trends, and more. LinkedIn is adding a filter to prevent group spamming and odd endorsements popping onto your page.

If you're in private practice and not on LinkedIn, you will miss out on a great amount of networking. Professional content consumption is on the rise. Over 1.5 million unique publishers actively use the LinkedIn Share button on their sites to send content into the LinkedIn platform. LinkedIn is accessed 91% of the time for professionally relevant content, compared to 64% of online news sites, 29% at Twitter, 27% at Facebook, and 16% at Google+.

Professional content covers subjects such as new research, breaking industry news, case studies (remembering HIPAA, of course), and career advice. It is brief and concise in length and produced by an industry leader.

Here is a list of mistakes, based on the work of Leanne Kennis (2012), commonly made by professionals on LinkedIn:

- Not having a profile photo, using an unprofessional photo, or using a poorly cropped photo.

- Not updating your contact information. People need to be able to reach you.

- Not completing your entire profile. Brand your profile by creating a custom URL, design a catchy headline, and list all experience related to your current profession.

- Not including a personalized message for the invitation to followers or for connections you would like to make. Use the boilerplate invitation and customize it to fit your needs.

- Not posting appropriate content. Content needs to be professional and relevant.

- Not proofreading your posts. Posts with misspellings, the wrong word, or other grammatical mistakes degrade your professionalism.

- Not contributing to the conversation.

- Not being selective about the connections you accept. Your connections are a reflection of who you are and what your practice represents.

- Not becoming a thought leader, the person with expertise in your field.

- Not helping others. Offer your expertise to people in your profession, answer questions in your LinkedIn network, and support projects and efforts advocated by your connections.

- Not starting a group around a professional topic, rather than just your company.

Pinterest

Pinterest, started in March 2010, allows users to save images and categorize them on different boards. It has grown from a site where viewers made "boards" with pictures of their hobbies, their favorite places, and cute kittens, to a 70 million user network with professionals marketing their practices. It drives more traffic to websites and blogs than YouTube, Google+, and LinkedIn combined. The website has proven especially popular among women. Starting as a by-invitation-only media site, Pinterest no longer requires a request or an invitation to join the site.

Social media expert, Beth Hayden, has authored the e-publication *Pinfluence: The Complete Guide to Marketing Your Business with Pinterest* (2013). Her website offers courses, newsletters, and blog posts on marketing your practice on Pinterest. These are fabulous resources if you choose Pinterest for your marketing plan.

Business pages on Pinterest can serve as a "virtual storefront" and can include prices of products and services. "Shopify tracked merchants in the U.S., Canada, the U.K., and Australia from September 2011 through April 2012. The sales figures showed that Pinterest users spent more money—an average of $80 per order—than customers who came through other networks like Facebook and Twitter" (Ross, 2012). In 2013, Pinterest introduced a new tool called 'Rich Pins.' These Pins allow you to add extra information right on the Pin. You can place a Pin on a map that has your business name, address, and phone number. You can use a Pin to link to articles. And you can include Pins with product information.

For business pages, use your business name, description, website address, and links to your other social media locations. Pin photos daily to keep your content fresh. Choose photos that reflect your practice values, ethics, and branding. Pins of professional content can also be added to your boards, and you'll want to add an "On Hover Pin It" button to your content, available with directions for use on Pinterest. Choose the best blogs, videos, and articles from colleagues and pin them to your boards. The best times to share new content are midday Thursday and Saturday morning. Provide unique information through ideas like coaching, book reviews, and Group Boards, justifying content with facts, quote comments (with permission, of course) from clients and events, and whatever methods you can come up with. Pinterest provides a statistics page that allows you to see a return for your effort.

Pinterest has a notification system that allows copyright holders to request that content be removed from the site. Because Pinterest allows users to transfer information, intellectual property rights come into play. In early May 2012, the site added automatic attribution of authors on images originating from other social media sites. Automatic attribution was also added for Pins from sites mirroring content on Flickr. At the same time, Flickr added a Pin shortcut to its share option menu to users who have not opted out of sharing their images (http://en.wikipedia.org/wiki/Pinterest).

Twitter

Twitter was released in July 2006 as an online social networking and microblogging site. It allows users to send and read short text messages (140 or less characters) called "tweets." Registered users can read and post tweets, but unregistered users can only read them. In 2013, Twitter handled 1.6 billion search queries each day.

If you would like to tweet about your private practice, choose a good Twitter "handle" or name. This can be your name, the name of your business, a variation of both, or an abbreviated version of either. Making your handle reflect your business is important. You'll want to post it (@name) on your website, in signature lines, and on your written materials. In your business marketing plan, have specific goals for tweeting, whether it is to announce new events, classes, point to your blog or a new video, or other business announcements. Create your Twitter profile with your business goals in mind, and be sure to include a link to your website. Hashtags are used to organize tweets around names, categories, topics, or themes. Use Twitter Search to view what others have tweeted about breastfeeding and other topics, to see who has tweeted about your business name, or to view what other similar professionals are tweeting.

The Twitter Help Center has an extensive number of informational articles on getting started; finding content related to your interests; managing your profile and account settings; how to interact with others; on-the-go apps for iPhones, Androids, and mobile phones; solutions to common issues; Twitter Rules and reporting violations; and Twitter Ads. It even contains information on what to do if you believe you've been hacked to protect your account and change your password.

YouTube

YouTube, a video sharing website, is the second largest search engine on the globe. It allows you to search for just about anything, including your favorite music video, how-to videos about any subject under the sun, and professional videos on healthcare matters. The videos tend to be short and very focused on the topic; think "quick step-by-step," rather than an hour of how-tos.

YouTube allows anyone to post videos. When you post, you are given the option to restrict views to only certain people or to post it publicly, allowing viewers to share it in a wide variety of venues. Lactation teaching videos abound on YouTube and include excellent ones on Reverse Pressure Softening, manual expression, pumping, supplementing baby at the breast, paced bottle feeding, cup feeding, and more. It is an excellent tool for demonstrations to mothers during consultations, hospital visits, or via email or online counseling.

YouTube was created in 2005. It underwent a major revamp in 2011, with a new homepage concentrating on channels, a new color palate, the video "Slam" voting contest, a "filter & explore" search option, a video editing feature, and the Copyright School to educate copyright offenders about their mistakes.

As of February 2011, YouTube had 490 million unique users worldwide per month, who racked up an estimated 92 billion page views each month (www.mashable.com). More than 3 billion videos are viewed per day, and users upload the equivalent of 240,000 full-length films every week. About 70% of YouTube traffic comes from outside the U.S. YouTube is localized in 25 countries through 43 languages, and the demographic is broad— mostly consisting of 18- to 54-year-olds.

Whether or not you add to the professional content materials on YouTube, you will want to spend some time on the website to investigate what is available in the lactation field.

When The Lactation Connection (TLC) Inc. began, social media was not really an option. The main push in my business plan was to build a website and keep it updated. At that time, hiring a professional to build an excellent website was either too expensive or they lacked knowledge about the special needs of a lactation consultant. I purchased my web domain and a website-building package. This was beneficial to get the website up and running, but required a tremendous amount of time and knowledge on my part. Email communications were the next addition to the business plan. Most communications with healthcare providers were done by regular postal methods or by faxing reports.

Today, though, the options are mind-boggling. With Breastfeeding Perspectives™, I am using LinkedIn, Pinterest, Twitter, and Facebook with good results. Many social media experts now offer free webinars to teach how to best market via social media, usually as a give-away for their own services (research the Beth Hayden presentations, for example). These can be very valuable for basic information and provide an example of a give-away product method that can be employed by private practice LCs. According to Porterfield, Khare, & Vahl (2011), a coupon or giveway is "great for attracting attention to your product, building brand awareness, or launching a product. Coupons and giveaways on Facebook are easily shared with friends; people love to get special deals." These types of promotions increase traffic to your website, participation in your online community, sharing among friends, and excitement about your services.

Private Practice Self-Check

How do you plan to reach new mothers through social media?

How will you make sure your social media dealings are professional?

How will you maintain the privacy and confidentiality of your clients when using social media?

Chapter Eleven. Advertising and Marketing

The toughest thing about success is that you've got to keep on being a success.

~Irving Berlin

Well-organized business owners have a written marketing plan, which includes sales, public relations, market research, advertising, media planning, customer support, and community involvement. You will notice that advertising is but a small part of marketing; the two are not synonymous. One simple definition of marketing could be everything you do to touch the consumer who will be using your services and products.

Advertising

In order to reach new clients and retain existing clients, you will need to advertise your services. This can be accomplished through radio and television ads, Internet ads, newspaper and magazine ads, flyers, brochures, emails, signage, direct mail, and/or other specific activities. In order to reach those who may be in need of your services, you will find using a combination of venues to be the best method. Advertising tends to be expensive, so plan for a sizable portion of your financial budget to be set aside for advertising.

Plan to track the effectiveness of your ads. Each new advertising campaign your practice produces should quantify the number of new leads, which of those leads became clients, the cost of each campaign, were there return clients, and whether you received referrals from existing clientele. Without this (and more) tracking, you will not ascertain which campaigns were successful and which should not be repeated. Determining the source of every new client will allow you to determine the effectiveness of each of your various advertising techniques.

How do you determine what media outlets you want to use to advertise? Begin by determining who you are trying to reach and study that population's habits. Will it be the educated new mother who can easily afford your services? Or will it be the well-insured patient? WIC clientele? Those who only want home visits? Those who will come to your office? Where do these potential clients receive their information and referrals for your services? Use media that targets the group you are looking to capture and know that media well. For example, if you decide to run a black and white ad in a local health magazine, spend time going through back issues of the magazine. Do the articles meet the tone of your private practice mission statement and the way you provide your services? Do your competitors advertise in the same magazine? Are there inappropriate advertisements in the magazine that would conflict with your mission?

Choose a medium that will keep your name and professional services in the forefront of new mothers' minds. Use a medium that primarily targets those to whom your message is aimed. And then hit that demographic over and over again. Frequency of advertising and allowing adequate time for the advertising to work are two secrets to a successful ad campaign. Stopping a particular campaign prematurely may have negative consequences; mothers need to see an ad multiple times in order to begin to trust in those services. Your ad, backed up with a referral from their physician or a friend, may mean a new client for your practice.

Avoid the shotgun approach—using many different media approaches for advertising. To many, this appears "needy" and desperate and may not portray the professionalism you desire for your services.

To determine which media is right for you, identify your number one objective. Is it to introduce your practice to the community? Introduce a new product to mothers? Establish your practice's position and dominance? Create a call to action? Once you have this figured out, plan to devote a substantial budgetary amount to your marketing campaign. If this medium is working and you have discretionary monies in your budget, beef up areas where you already advertise to heighten the effect.

Any ads should project the professionalism of your practice; do not substitute amateurish efforts in your advertising, which can decrease the professional image you are trying to project. A brochure in development, for example, may benefit from a professional printing service for design and printing rather than a color copy from your printer. This is your reputation being submitted to the public venue, and nothing should be more important than your reputation. The public makes judgments about what they don't know yet based on what they do know; they will judge your practice and you by your marketing materials and advertisements.

As an example of what not to do, I will share the excitement I felt when a local radio station called to "personally" request that I submit a short spot on breastfeeding for airwave play on their station. As a new private practitioner, I had little knowledge of the slick marketing procedures used to garner business in various avenues. Of course, I agreed without doing much research as to return on investment or having this outlay of money within my business plan. I was only thinking about the airtime and marketing of the practice. It was a terrific three-minute piece that actually used the word "breastfeeding" on the air! But it produced no new leads and was much more expensive than I would have normally budgeted for. That proved a hard-learned lesson.

One marketing ploy that was highly successful was marketing a one-hour lunchtime education feature to local physician office staff, called "Milk and Cookies." When each free session was booked, I stopped by the best bakery in town, got fresh chocolate-chip cookies, and provided their choice of inservice topics for one hour. A portion of that time always included what TLC Inc. provided for their clients, how to access help through TLC Inc., what reports were provided to each healthcare provider by TLC Inc., and how to contact the practice with professional questions and needs. Within one month of advertising this service, I was providing three to five inservices each week and receiving referrals of mothers with problems from the providers given the additional education.

Marketing

The marketing methods lactation professionals use to promote their individual practices can also serve to educate and inform the public about lactation issues, treatment options, and the value of the service. The final goal should be to refrain from harming or manipulating the public, using ethical means to get the word out about your practice.

Marketing includes not only advertising, but a broader range of activities for getting your services known to all those who can impact your target market. Target not only new mothers, but their healthcare providers, insurance providers, family members, other lactation professionals, and those who would be referring new mothers to your services. Decide what it is that you provide best to your target population, and then make sure all of your advertising and marketing ideas are consistent with that message. Market your practice as close to your inherent talents, best skills, and passion as possible. You want to love what you do each and every day. The following suggestions will help you develop a good marketing plan.

Evidence-Based Marketing

Use evidence-based marketing by including proven strategies, a well-designed marketing plan, effective implementation, and evaluation of the results. Without any one of these components, you are not capturing the full potential of your marketing.

Update Regularly

Update your marketing plan on a regular basis, say every three to six months. Even very effective marketing goals and plans can become outdated and may need regular review and refreshing.

Goals and Strategies

Use clear goals and strategies to carry out your marketing plan. Goals are specific and quantifiable, strategies support goals, and tactics implement the strategies. Use a timeline for completion of each goal, strategy, and tactic.

Customer Service and Satisfaction

Provide excellence in customer service and satisfaction, from how the initial telephone or Internet contact is answered to making sure the client is happy and satisfied with the end product or service they received from you. You can develop a format to survey satisfaction after the client has been seen, whether it be a postage-paid card that can be filled out and mailed later or an online survey to have clients share their experience with the service. Determine in advance how you will handle complaints or client dissatisfaction. It should apply across the board to all clientele and be evidenced in your Policy Notebook.

Helpful Expert

Become the helpful expert in your ongoing relationship with the public. This continual promotion of your practice and expertise will allow others to see you in a positive light and will build your reputation. This takes consistent and intentional efforts.

Use of press releases to the local media (newspaper, radio, and television stations) takes skill and tenacity. These may be provided by postal mail, electronic distribution from your own media list with the aid of a distribution service, faxing short releases and press advisories, or overnight delivery of full color press kits for an impressive impact. Since media is often inundated with press requests, inventory your information: Is it newsworthy, does it meet the audience of that particular outlet, is it providing something new or something old in a new way, and is it timely with tie-ins to current events?

Participate in interviews with the local media to promote your expertise in the field. When you receive a journalist or producer request, be ready with the information immediately, since they often work under tight deadlines. Remember to be flexible, available, courteous, and provide them with plenty of background materials. This is a relationship-building move with the media, just as you provide to your clients. Be aware of the "spin" of the story for which you are being quoted. You may not receive rights to review the information prior to it being aired or going to press.

Writing for publications from newspapers to professional journals is an excellent way to become a subject matter expert. Keep your writing educational and helpful rather than self-promoting. Give suggestions, new ideas, how-tos, warnings, resources, and advice. Always include a biographical note with your name, address, and telephone number.

Professional speaking is one of the most effective means to generate referrals and to make your practice known in the community. You may want to provide lectures, free talks, brown bag lunch presentations, seminars, classes, radio interviews, television show interviews, workshops, or speeches to civic or religious organizations. You can include in these speeches successful case studies (HIPPA compliant, of course) where you were able to help someone against all odds; personal stories about your own struggles and how you overcame them; and/or discussion of your moral, ethical, or mission values that guide your work with mothers. Having those listening feel connected to you is a strong goal of speaking.

Being active in your community shows passion and caring and can build your reputation as well. Make sure you maximize your efforts in involvement by providing your professional skills for the benefit of the community members. Provision of things like a donation of your services for a fundraising auction, involvement on a community Board of Directors, participation in healthcare committees, giving a free speech at the passing of a breastfeeding-friendly ordinance or dedication of a new pumping facility–think outside the typical marketing box.

Community Relationships

Plan relationships to build marketing in the community, which will grow into very successful networks, opportunities, and client referrals over time. Make a plan to connect with those who can provide referrals to your practice and expect to receive a 10% return on your time and efforts. For example, if you plan to meet a new professional each week for one full year, that gives you 50 new contacts. A 10% return would result in five contacts who become good referral sources. Think outside the lactation community–counselors, nail technicians, daycare providers, financial planners, spas, printers, baby-store owners, massage therapists, health food store owners, family dentists, yoga studio owners. Then add those from the healthcare industry, such as midwives, doulas, childbirth educators, obstetricians, pediatricians, family practice physicians, mother-to-mother support group leaders, hospital birthing centers, infant chiropractors. The list is endless!

Branding

Branding is vital to your image. If you are the only private practice lactation consultant in your area, branding might not be as important. However, if your competitors are active, you need to have your community and clients clearly hear and understand your message...how are you different and better than anyone else in town.

Branding is your practice's "personality" and should be defined prior to spending any money on advertising or marketing. Your brand is not your logo or your business card. It should be what your practice stands for, what it is known for by the public, the promise you provide to the community. You should create an image in the mind of your potential clients.

Strategies that can help create your brand include:

- **Determine your audience.** The wider population you wish to reach needs to be defined, their needs and desires identified, and their struggles and challenges understood. Within that wider audience, find your niche, the clients who will benefit most from the services you will provide. As your practice grows, you will find new niches to reach, along with the services needed to do so.

- **Discover your brand values.** What is the passion and purpose behind your business, the inspiration for the creation of the practice, what value can you provide to your clients? These values should be authentic, earnest, enthusiastic declarations of what you want your brand to portray. Don't compare yourself to the competition, but keep the wording and branding positive, focusing on your values and benefits for the families you aim to assist.

- Above all, **be honest.** Communicate with respect and authenticity at every opportunity. The more you know and can effectively communicate about your practice, the higher the impact on your success. Treat everyone with honesty, respect, and genuineness, and word will spread far and wide that your practice can be trusted to provide the best service.

- Brand for **recognition and impression.** Your business needs a brand that is designed for uniqueness, evoking emotion within those in your niche. Don't skimp on the budget for this aspect; plan to hire a quality graphic artist to brand your website, logo, business cards, brochures, stationary, forms, and emails. Have your brand become instantly recognizable to reinforce the values you intend to portray.

- **Be consistent** again and again. Capitalize on your brand values, the impressive design, and your intimate knowledge of client needs with consistency at every opportunity. All communications, be they email, regular postal mail, website, telephone, or in-person, need to reinforce your message, product, and service.

- Do you use **color** or not? There is an entire field of psychology related to the study of color, a truly fascinating study of human behavior. However, culture, experiences, personal preference, and context all affect how color is perceived by the consumer. Colors can affect how the consumer views the personality of the brand you are presenting, so some research is in order. The consumer reaction to the color is more important than the specific color. For example, brown fosters feelings of ruggedness, purple fosters sophistication, red excitement, green calm, white clean and calm. It is generally accepted that men prefer bright, bold colors, while women prefer softer colors. This is yet another reason to work with a graphic artist to design the best branding for your practice; an investment that will pay off in the long run.

Blog Away

You might consider having a blog on your website where you can regularly write articles that speak to those in your niche. Blog posts are generally 300 to 500 words, provided at least weekly, and allow you to tag in order for search engines to pick up the post in searches. Don't let the fact that your current website doesn't provide a blog keep you from blogging. Free sites can be set up at wordpress.com, typepad.com, or blogspot.com. Blog details are described more fully in Chapter Ten.

Market Online

Use social media for marketing, such as Pinterest, FaceBook, LinkedIn, Twitter, Google Plus, Yahoo! Buzz, MySpace, Stumbleupon, Technorati, YouTube, Yelp, webinars, online newsletters, guest blogs, regular email blasts, expert articles, and anything else you can delve into. Be aware, though, that dealing with all markets might present more work for you than desired, as well as taking time away from client consultations. Consider tackling one social media market and become proficient at it before entering a second, third, or fourth market (see Chapter Ten for more information on social media).

Marketing Plan

As a new IBCLC in private practice, it is easy to get drawn into yet one more venue for marketing just because it sounds good at the time. Your biggest challenge in a small business is to simplify and make your marketing plan to guide your efforts and budget. Remind yourself regularly that protecting your professional image is your number one priority. When you receive a request to enter a new market, ask yourself: Does this help me, does this hurt me, and does it have a large or small effect? If the new venue is hurtful to your practice or has little to no effect, say NO immediately. If it helps or has a large effect, ask yourself: Does it fit with my current budget, available time, expenses, and marketing plan?

Many marketing professionals use a circular formula for creating a marketing plan. They use the acronym RACE, which stands for research, action planning, communication of the plan, and execution/evaluation. Each portion of the process is a part of the previous process. Research reviews evaluation of previous efforts. Successful efforts are included in the action plan. The action plan is communicated, which leads to execution. Part of the execution includes evaluating the effectiveness of the plan. The evaluation provides research for future plans. And on and on. Templates for marketing plans are freely available online and provide a great start to the RACE procedure.

Competition

Competition between colleagues often implies that there is a finite limit to the number of clients who would benefit from the help of a lactation consultant. Remember that many mothers are not getting the help they need to overcome breastfeeding problems for a variety of reasons. They may be under the impression that as a mother, they should be able to solve the problem themselves. Or their problem could go undiagnosed. They could have been seen by a less-practiced lactation provider (or even someone without credentialing and training) and believe that since that person could not solve their problem, all providers are the same and unable to assist them. There is a vast, untapped population of mothers having breastfeeding problems who could benefit from your services. Target that population and don't fret over the numbers of mothers being seen by your "competition."

Clientele

Keep track of past and current clients by email. You can send regular email communications via e-zine, e-newsletter, article of the month, announcements of new services or products, happy mother's day or other holiday celebrations. Remember, though, that you must have their permission to do this; no spamming allowed. Design a quick and easy survey for past and current clients, asking them for ideas on what services and support they would like to see added to your practice. Do not assume you know what they want; ask them!

Thank You

When was the last time you received a thank you note from a company with whom you did business? Not many can say that it happens frequently, but when it does, what feelings are stirred about that company? Make it your rule to send a thank you note to everyone who refers a new client to you, whether they are the physician, the grandmother, another client, or the local hospital lactation consultant. Be specific in your thanks, it feels so much more valuable to the recipient. Remember that it's about them and not about you. And most importantly, in this day and age of text messages, emails, and Internet communication, revive the old-school method of a handwritten note sent by postage mail. The meaning and impression to the recipient are irreplaceable.

In an online interview, Dr. Katharine Hansen (2014) was asked, "What's the best format for a thank-you note? Should it be a typed business letter or a handwritten social note?" Her answer? "Studies show it doesn't matter. The important thing is doing it. Tailor your letter to the culture of the company and the relationship you established with the person who interviewed you. If you feel the interviewer and the company call for a formal business letter, send that. If your rapport with the interviewer dictate a more personal touch, send a handwritten note."

Customer Loyalty Program

Develop and implement a customer loyalty program. New customers are the growth of your practice, but you must ensure return business from current and long-standing clients. They deserve VIP treatment. Having a loyal client see products or services for which they paid full price discounted to entice new clients will cause ill will and potential loss of that loyal client. Think about offering exclusive programs, deals, or specials specifically geared to your most loyal clients.

Experienced LCs Share

Please share at least three marketing ideas that have worked well for you and your practice. The marketing tools used by IBCLCs varied from practice to practice. Presented here are the tools from the IBCLCs themselves:

- Website, which must be up-to-date, eye catching, and listed on search engines.

- Business cards and brochures for pediatric and obstetric offices.

- Notebooks of breastfeeding information, along with marketing information for the private practice given to physicians and birthing centers to place in their waiting rooms.

- Laminated weight loss charts and prescription pads for a lactation consult provided to pediatricians for referral to the practice.

- Networking is a must, since most of the clients come from word-of-mouth.

- Exhibiting at local conferences for lactation, nursing, physicians, WIC, doulas, mother-to-mother support groups, babywearing, midwifery, and childbirth education.

- Faxing consult reports to the client's pediatrician and obstetrician/midwife— always. One IBCLC recommends making the goal to herself to have it faxed by midnight of the day of the consult. Another would not cash the check or run the credit card until the reports were sent.

- Offering lunch-and-learns to pediatric practices. One IBCLC called the 30-minute presentation "Milk & Cookies" and provided fresh baked cookies for the staff.

- File folders left with the mother after each consult, with her clinical care plan and marketing materials for her to share with others.

- Taking goodies (candy, fruit basket, cookies, muffins) to the OB and Pediatric offices; not at Christmas or Holiday times, but during World Breastfeeding Week. This allows a lack of competition from all the other companies that provide holiday treats, and time to meet the staff.

- Ask your client to TELL her OB and Pediatrician that the services she received from you were worth the cost.

- Newsletters, either for mothers or for healthcare professionals. Monthly contact with the providers keeps your name and branding in front of them, and providing good breastfeeding education in the newsletter helps to keep it in the office rather than being thrown away.

- Creation of a business Facebook page is helpful to reach the 20- and 30-something mothers who rely on technology and on the referrals of others for your services.

- Sponsoring events for the local doulas, mother-to-mother groups, breastfeeding coalitions, childbirth educators, and mother support groups help to get your name out to the public.

- Blog, blog, blog!

- Become a lactation media expert for your local newspapers, television, and radio stations.

- Write articles for other organizations.

- Have your practice information present on all local hospital referral lists.

Private Practice Self-Check

How will you advertise your new business?

This advertising cost will cost approximately:

How will you market your new business?

This marketing will cost approximately:

How will you determine the effectiveness of your advertising and marketing efforts?

Chapter Twelve. Self-Care for the Business Owner

Be gentle with yourself. You are a child of the universe, no less than the trees and the stars. In the noisy confusion of life, keep peace in your soul.

~Max Ehrmann

Those that enter the profession of lactation support often do so because they are passionate about mothers and babies. They are nurturers, caregivers, tenders, and providers. Self-care generally falls to the end of the "to-do" list for these personalities. However, to be the best lactation consultant, business owner, family member, and caregiver, you absolutely must take care of yourself.

Stress

In ancient times, the body's physical response to stress was an essential adaptation for meeting natural threats to health and existence. Even today, the stress response can be an asset for raising levels of performance during critical events, such as a sports competition, an important meeting, giving a speech, or a crisis situation. If stress becomes prolonged, however, all parts of the body's stress apparatus, including the brain, heart, lungs, blood vessels, and muscles, become chronically over-activated. This may produce physical or psychological damage over time. Research studies have suggested that chronic stress can lead to depression, anxiety, heart disease, stroke, susceptibility to infection, immune disorders, cancer, gastrointestinal problems, eating disorders, diabetes, pain, sleep disturbances, sexual and reproductive dysfunctions, memory and concentration difficulties, and learning disorders (Parkes, 2004).

Stress can have positive or negative effects on an individual. Acute stress has been defined as intermittent and short-lived, whereas chronic stress tends to last prolonged periods of time, often several weeks or longer. Habituation to chronic stress is possible and ideal, but failure to do so can lead to detrimental effects on the body, including sleep disturbances and changes in pain thresholds (Steckler, 2001). The occurrence of stress is dependent on the degree to which the individual perceives environmental demands as threatening, challenging, or harmful. Grant et al. (2003) suggested a better definition of stress as, "environmental events or chronic conditions that objectively threaten the physical and/or psychological health or well-being of individuals."

Hans Selye, considered the father of stress theory, was the first to suggest that the body initially responds to stress with a physiological activation of defense systems (Elsyek, 1936). A resistance phase follows, during which the stress is to be resolved. If unsuccessful, the body may experience exhaustion. Activation that endures beyond the resistance state is hypothesized to cause disease.

The stress response is characterized by increases in glucose levels, heart rate, and blood pressure and decreases in feeding and reproduction (Steckler, 2001). Chronic stress leads to destruction and atrophy of neurons, decreased short-term and contextual memory, and poor regulation of endocrine response to stress (McEwen, 1998).

Hypertension is one long-term outcome linked to chronic stress. Normally, acute stress results in an increase of blood pressure and cardiac output and a decrease of total peripheral resistance. Chronic stress-induced high blood pressure and increased heart rate, in time, lead to the development of coronary artery disease and are causal factors in the development of increased cardiovascular risks, obesity, insulin resistance, and hypertension (Schwartz et al., 2003; Hjemdahl, 2002). Central (abdominal) obesity is associated with higher systemic vascular resistance during stress. Both skeletal muscle and skin vasodilation responses are impaired, suggesting decreased beta-adrenergic responsiveness, insulin resistance, increased activity of the renin-angiotensin system, and increased levels of pro-inflammatory cytokines (Narkiewicz, 2002).

Inflammation has been linked to many diseases. Stress decreases the immune system's capacity to respond effectively. Subsequently, the inflammatory process flourishes and has been implicated in poor wound healing, blunted responses to immunization, and to a host of opportunistic diseases. Increased risk for upper respiratory infection, acceleration in the progression of coronary artery disease, decreased activity of natural killer cells, and exacerbation in the course of autoimmune disorder have been noted in the chronically stressed.

Chronic stress in humans can create multiple health behaviors that put them at greater health risk, including poorer nutrition, poorer sleep, higher use of alcohol, tobacco, and drugs, and less exercise.

Stress creates sustained autonomic nervous system arousal affecting both rapid eye movement (REM) and non-REM sleep, reflected in the amount of wakefulness during sleep and in the lower number of delta counts, which indicate deep sleep. There is also a psychophysiological factor of insomnia, including elevations in body and skin temperature, increased muscle tone, higher metabolic activity, and elevated heart rate.

High levels of stress produce increased gastric acid production, an inhibition of gastric emptying time, and an impairment of the diaphragmatic portion of the lower esophageal sphincter mechanism by stress-related shallow breathing patterns. This exacerbates symptoms of gastrointestinal tract disorders, including gastroesophageal reflux disease and chronic severe heartburn.

Compassion Fatigue

As lactation consultants, we have dedicated our lives to empathizing with the mothers we serve–caring for them and providing help to correct problems. We are 'fixers." As such, LCs are especially prone to burnout, a natural consequence of caring for clients who are in pain, suffering, or traumatized. The current term for burnout of caregivers is compassion fatigue or secondary traumatic stress, secondary stress syndrome, or secondary victimization. The term, compassion fatigue, was created by Carla Johnson in 1992 after noting the loss of ability to nurture in nurses and emergency medical workers caring for patients suffering severe illness and traumatic events.

Compassion fatigue shows manifestations of physical, emotional, and spiritual exhaustion and is a progressive state of emotional turbulence. Lactation consultants are not immune to the feelings experienced by the mothers they assist, often leading to emotional exhaustion. As the private practice clientele increase in numbers, many LCs do not have (or do not take) time to recover from the emotional overload experienced. Those who do not recognize and/or cope with the symptoms of compassion fatigue are often impeded in their ability to provide effective and nurturing care to their clients.

What are the symptoms of compassion fatigue in a lactation consultant?

- Withdrawal from friends, family, and other loved ones
- A loss of passion for working with mothers and babies
- Loss of interest in activities previously found to be enjoyable
- Feeling depressed, irritable, hopeless, helpless
- Changes in appetite, weight, or both
- Changes in sleep patterns
- More frequent illness
- Loss of energy to be consistently productive
- Lack of satisfaction in your job
- Feelings of wanting to hurt yourself or those you care for
- Emotional and physical exhaustion
- Excessive use of caffeine to maintain constant energy levels

- Use of alcohol, tobacco, or drugs to feel better or to blunt feelings

- Unexplained headaches, backaches, or other physical complaints

Multiple factors can increase the potential for compassion fatigue. Not being able to separate yourself from the plight of your client–taking on the decision of the mother as a personal victory or loss is unhealthy. The role of the LC is to provide evidence-based information and assistance to each mother and baby, and enable them to make the decision that is appropriate for them. Here's a helpful reminder to do this: Put a Q-tip® cotton swab on your computer monitor to remind yourself to "Quit Taking It Personally"…the accornym is QTip!

As caregivers, lactation consultants expect their interventions and involvement to improve the health of the client. This could potentially be an unrealistic expectation, since on occasion the situation may not improve for the breastfeeding mother and baby. You will find the client who needs your "permission" to stop breastfeeding, you may experience negative outcomes you did not anticipate, or you may have to refer the client to someone more experienced than yourself. These are not often what LCs expect in their assistance of clients.

Many caregivers become frustrated by a lack of money, time, skills, or resources to effectively plan and implement the care they desire to provide. This lack of control can escalate the feelings of stress.

Trying to be everything to everyone is an unreasonable demand to place upon yourself. You cannot be "on duty" 24 hours a day, seven days a week; no one can. Keep reminding yourself that it is NOT your responsibility to provide exclusive care to every breastfeeding mother and baby in your area.

Strive to maintain balance between your professional work and your home life. When you identify so strongly with the passionate work you provide that you lack a reasonable balance, you may be more likely to experience burnout. The demands of family, especially with young children, cannot be put aside. Remember, everything in moderation.

Experienced LCs Share

What do you wish you had known prior to going into private practice?

Setting boundaries appears to be difficult for most in the caring profession of lactation–wanting to assist every client that called, being available 24/7, rearranging other engagements to see an "emergency" client, and being available at times when no one calls for assistance. The hard work involved in being a business person, as well as a lactation consultant, was mentioned by all respondents. There needs to be a continual effort to stay on top of the business paperwork and reporting, and much of that time is not reimbursable. Time spent returning telephone calls, setting appointments, answering emails, filing, reporting to healthcare providers, figuring and filing tax paperwork, researching answers to breastfeeding questions, and much more is not usually billable time.

The topic of emotional tolls was described in several ways: being too invested in the outcome of clients, long-term relationships with mothers over weeks, months and even years, the high amount of energy devoted to the passion of the practice, and being overwhelmed with the fast growth of the practice were highlighted.

Taking Care of Yourself

There are various areas of self-care that can keep you healthy, happy, spiritually connected, at peace, and able to provide what is needed to family, friends, and clientele.

Physical Care

Assess your diet and nutrition. Do you eat regularly? Do you eat healthy foods? Or do you skip meals or grab an unhealthy alternative because it is quick and easy?

Do you exercise regularly to keep your body in tip-top shape? Exercise can be whatever makes you feel great–yoga, running, walking, biking, hiking, spinning, swimming, sports, or dancing. Even walking the dog is exercise. Aim for thirty minutes each day, at least five days a week for the best health and stress relief. It must be a form of exercise that you don't detest engaging in, that you won't put off until tomorrow because there "just isn't time for it."

Take care of yourself medically. Do you take time off of work when ill? Do you get regular medical check-ups? Do you keep on top of your prevention care, such as routine breast self-exams, mammograms, and pap smears? These are all important.

Take vacations regularly, get a massage, sleep to meet your body's needs, and wear clothes you really like! Learn breathing exercises that increase tension relief in your muscles and wake up the brain with oxygenation.

Psychological Care

Psychologically, you need time for self-reflection, meditation, journaling, and/or "mental health days," with time away from work. Read literature that does not have anything to do with lactation. Go to a concert, art show, theater production, sports event that will help you relax and provide a change of pace for your mind and soul. Most importantly, learn to say no to those obligations that do not serve your values and life mission.

Recharge Your Battery

Because you are a caregiver, learn to recharge your own battery to preserve your emotional health. Spend time with those whose company you enjoy, with those you love, and those who make you laugh. Give yourself affirmations and praise on a daily basis. When you find yourself outraged over a social injustice, funnel that energy into action with letter writing, donations, marches, protests, or other creative outlets. Pursue a hobby that has little or nothing to do with breastfeeding and private practice, and jump into it with a passion. You might not need to choose a new hobby...what did you abandon when your practice began? It's still there, awaiting your return, be it golf, quilting, antiquing, baking, learning another language, or any of a thousand different options.

Humor

Make others...and yourself...laugh. Humor keeps us sane even during the most stressful of times. Laughter releases endorphins, those feel-good hormones that elevate mood and reduce stress.

Attitude

Maintain the right attitude by being optimistic, allowing yourself to not be a perfectionist (in fact, become a "recovering perfectionist"!), being mindful, letting go of anger, and having fun each day.

Spirituality

Connect with your spirituality using reflection, meditation, prayer, singing. Go out into nature, be open to inspiration, find meaning in everyday experiences. Find a spiritual community with which to be involved. Provide yourself with small things, such as a daily inspirational quote, aromatherapy, music, or even petting your favorite cat or dog.

Life Mission Statement

Is it time that you reviewed (or even developed for the first time) your own life mission statement? Take a day or even an entire weekend and write a declaration of purpose for your life. By stepping back and looking at your life as a whole, you may find that the current life stressors are put into proper perspective. Set up a morning ritual to begin your day. It might include sitting in a sunny spot with a cup of tea and a good book, doing yoga, journaling, or prayer. Whatever the routine, it will begin your day with focus and purpose. Take care of yourself instead of bursting out of bed, wolfing down something for a so-called breakfast, and storming out the door with a high level of stress to begin the day.

Relationships

Don't forget to schedule time for your partner and children. Make dates with your best friends for a night out, lunch, or breakfast together, or a routine telephone check-in. Allow others to do for you, instead of being the expert or in charge of everything. Increase those in your social circle outside of lactation. And most importantly, ask for help when you need it.

Take a Break

During your official workday, be sure to take a break for lunch or just to step outside for a few moments of sunshine. Set aside quiet time for completion of tasks that need your full attention. Identify projects or tasks that are exciting, rewarding, and provide you with pleasure. Set limits with clients, co-workers, and others who might demand more of you than you are able to give.

Workspace

Arrange your workspace for comfort, organization, visual pleasure, and to soothe and feed your soul. This can be accomplished with de-cluttering, music, aromatherapy, or inspiring photos.

Peer Support

Get involved with a peer support group. When you are in private practice, many times you will find a spirit of competition in your city from others in the same business. Go online to join with other private practitioners to be able to garner support and ideas, vent frustrations, and receive feedback.

Mindfulness

The popular concept of mindfulness has been found to help caregivers reduce stress and anxiety, decrease pain levels, increase inner peace, let go of negative thoughts, increase feelings of self-esteem, and relax the busyness of the mind. Mindfulness meditation is moment-to-moment awareness, being fully awake, and involves being here for the moments of our lives without striving or judging. It is a relaxed state of awareness that observes both your inner world of thoughts, feelings, and sensations, and the outer world of constantly changing phenomena, without trying to control anything. Dr. Jon Kabat-Zinn developed the Mindfulness Based Stress Reduction (MBSR) concept and program at the University of Massachusetts Medical Center in 1979. Since its inception, MBSR has evolved into a common form of complementary medicine to address various health issues (Kabat-Zinn, 2014) and is offered in over 200 medical centers, hospitals, and clinics worldwide. Classes to learn the art of mindfulness are offered at the Mindfulness Center in Massachusetts, as well as in many other cities.

Let's close this chapter on self-care with a wonderful quote:

The perfect no-stress environment is the grave. When we change our perception we gain control. The stress becomes a challenge, not a threat. When we commit to action, to actually doing something rather than feeling trapped by events, the stress in our life becomes manageable.

~ Greg Anderson

Private Practice Self-Check

What are ways you can decrease stress in your life?

How can you improve your physical health? Eat healthy meals? Exercise more? Get enough sleep?

What will you add to your life to improve your psychological health?

Chapter Thirteen. What I Would Have Done Differently

A collection of mistakes is called experience and experience is the key to success.

~ Unknown

In the final question of the survey, I asked the LC respondents to share things they would not repeat if they were starting their practice over again. Their suggestions and wishes, quoted here, were very revealing:

"If I could afford it, I would set up a private office and have clients come to me."

"I would spend more time being mentored by an experienced private practice LC."

"I would not overinvest my time without compensation."

"I would not get an outside office."

"I would not be as free with sharing of practice information. Recently, I had several people take advantage of that generosity and open their own practice utilizing many of my plans. I was disappointed that I had shared freely, and even more, that I did not see it coming. This does not create camaraderie."

"I would not include a follow-up consult in my initial fee, as it was very difficult to manage and it was never brief."

"Being a sole proprietorship is exhausting and unpredictable. I would recommend a partnership so that expenses and plans could be shared, although that presents different issues."

"I would not be so shy about asserting myself as a knowledgeable healthcare team member and find more ways to network with physicians."

"I would want to understand business better or to hire it out for things like filling out and filing taxes at the federal, state, and local levels."

"Having a better computer background would be helpful or pay for services like website design, creating software, designing and printing forms and handouts."

"Not get sucked into telephone conversations, as you end up giving a consult for free and it prevents the client from scheduling an appointment."

"Spend the money for a logo design and trademark it. Make it something that can be seen in color or black and white so that printing and copying are easier."

"Find a way to barter services."

"I would make a budget to help divide the small amounts of income at first and be able to pay all expenses. Get in a habit of saving a portion of the pump rental income monthly that will help with making the large rental agreement payment at the first of the year."

"Do not print your prices on anything that could remain in circulation for a long time. Rather publish those prices on your website."

"Put a date on everything you print to enable identification for review and revision."

"Have a policy book for your practice."

"I would not have delved into the rental and retail sides of the practice so blindly."

"I would have done better research on credit card machine feasibility for my small business. I ended up paying more for the machine than I accrued in charges. Better options and Paypal are now prevalent."

"Having a separate telephone line is necessary; do not use your home phone number. Cell phones make this a much easier option now."

"I would spend more time on marketing materials for the practice rather than the hand-outs used for education."

"Set better boundaries regarding delivery of services. I let people off the hook regarding time of day of service delivery, payment schedules, and more. In every case, I was left holding the bag, spending my time to help them and not getting compensated. I now have a firm policy and schedule, charge people if they do not show for the consult or cancel their appointment late, and make strict payment arrangements."

"I would not spend the time and energy to become a provider with insurance companies. They withhold or deny payments for the smallest and worst reasons. I never saw any volume and had only big headaches trying to collect the money due me. They have tried, and continue to do so, to get me to discount services provided. My clients have always gotten reimbursement for my services."

"Be careful about ordering high volumes on inventory to get a price reduction. I have gotten stuck with unsalable or outdated items in such cases."

"Take an accounting course; this would have better prepared me for the financial management portion of the practice. Financial Peace University offers money management training. The course is inexpensive and available all over the U.S. I highly recommend taking it prior to opening your practice."

"I had a business partner twice. In both instances, the 'divorce' was costly and painful. I now remain independent, but partner with others who have their own businesses via contractual relationships."

"I will say that the biggest mistake that people make is thinking that being a business person is easy. The skills required for clinical practice are NOT the same as those required to run a business, and the ethics of either can conflict with the other. One has to have thick skin and a good business head to make it work. One also has to be very, very clear about the boundaries and must be able to work the ethical aspect on both fronts. I recommend anyone choosing to go into business for themselves take courses through the Small Business Administration before starting up a practice. Knowing what you need to have skills in is useful before setting out on a course of action only to find that you messed up because you didn't know better."

"In the early years of practice, paying a fee to be listed on other community and professional websites was a waste of money."

"I am extremely careful about offering pumps new to the lactation market, as there have been several that have not been good pumps."

"Having a partner who was not knowledgeable about business operations or respectful of paying bills before drawing a paycheck was detrimental to my practice. It's hard to find someone where you think alike about every aspect of business, but it's important if you are going to have a partner. I know the pains of a partnership gone bad, and I've learned when it comes to money, everything must be spelled out in writing, and even then it can go sour. I personally would never have a business partner again. I run my business with integrity and common sense. It is mine and I don't have to make excuses for anyone else. If things are not done right, I can blame myself and hold myself accountable to make things right."

These comments, suggestions, ideas, and advice are invaluable for consideration by the new IBCLC who is contemplating opening a private practice. We can all learn from the experiences and mistakes of those who have gone before us.

Private Practice Self-Check

Which of these suggestions will you consider when setting up your business?

Chapter Fourteen. Putting It All Together!

Success is not final, failure is not fatal: it is the courage to continue that counts.

~ Winston Churchill

Business Plan

Having a business plan is the first step in making your dream a reality. It helps you outline your business in an organized fashion. It gives you a map of how you will set up your business and where you want your business to go. It is a working document that needs to be updated annually or any time you make changes in your goals or operating procedures. A good business plan spells out who the company is, what it does, how goals are accomplished, and where the business is headed in the next specified time periods. Many small businesses operate on a three-to-five year business plan with regular review.

A basic business plan includes:

- **Executive Summary:** A brief overview of your business to include a description of your services and products, and how they fill a need.

- **Background:** How your company will be set up legally, who the owners are, what your mission statement is, where your business will be located, who the target market is.

- **Market Analysis:** Number of women giving birth in your community, number breastfeeding, what lactation services exist in your community, what services are needed, the growth potential for your company.

- **Strategical Operations:** How you are going to operate, what services you will provide, how you will provide them, who will provide back-up, what products will you sell, will you have a partner or partners, will you employ any staff.

- **Marketing:** How you will market your products and services, how you will get the word out about your business to the general public and to your target market, will you use paid advertising, will you use social media, will you use other forms of marketing–health fairs, interviews on radio, TV, newspapers, etc.

- **Finance:** How you will finance your business, how much you will charge for your services, how much you will charge for your products, what accounting method you will use, and how your practice will be profitable.

- **Appendix:** Back-up information for the different sections.

Writing Goals

Effective goals are important in getting your new business up and running. What date do you want to start your business? What do you need to do before that date to be able to open your doors for business?

Michael Hyatt, professional speaker, consultant, and author of "Platform: Get Noticed in a Noisy World," reports that people who write down their goals accomplish significantly more than those who do not write their goals (www.michaelhyatt.com).

A goal is a general statement about a desired outcome to be accomplished within a designated time frame. Goals should describe accomplishments rather than activities.

The acronym S.M.A.R.T. is frequently used in business to set effective goals:

Specific: Your goal should clearly describe what you want to accomplish in setting up your business, why it is important to set up your business, and how you intend to accomplish setting up your business. You need to address who, what, when, where, and why in your goal, and use action verbs (create, design, develop, implement, produce).

Measurable: To make your goal measurable, include a plan with targets and milestones that you can use to keep on track. Focus on using actions words.

Achievable: To make your goal attainable, it should be realistic. Include a plan that breaks your overall goal into smaller, more manageable action steps that use available resources to keep within the set timeframe. Start with an action verb (begin, run, finish, eliminate) rather than a to-be verb (am, be, have). Objectives should be within your control and influence; although it might be a stretch for you, it should still be something that you can achieve. Suggestion: Add your goal and action steps to a white board in your office as a daily reminder of what you need to do to get your business up and running.

Relevant: Your action steps should be relevant to getting your business up and running. As you set additional goals, ask yourself why they are important and how they will help your business achieve its objectives? Keep your goals based on current realities and conditions for your service area.

Time-based: An effective time-based goal is limited by a defined period of time and includes specific timelines for each step of the process. Writing a goal without a timeline will result in not accomplishing what you originally set out to do.

Here is an example of SMART goal setting:

Not SMART: Keep the practice website up-to-date.

SMART: Research updates and new material on breastfeeding for the website on the first Friday of each month; publish this new material by the following Friday. Each time new material is posted, review the current website content for other material that is out-of-date and delete/archive that material.

Write down your goals for your business and make time to review them regularly to assess your progress. Putting your intentions in writing will assist you in setting things in motion. Regular review of the goals, whether daily, weekly, or monthly, will keep you on target. As new items arise, add them to your action steps. Look at the big picture to keep yourself focused on the endpoint. And always set an end date for each goal; open-ended goals often mean slower progress, as there is no urgency or time pressure to get you moving!

Have you included in your business plan an objective to keep up with the ever-changing lactation field? What about keeping up with the small business industry?

Private Practice Self-Check

Business Plan

Executive Summary:

Give a brief overview of your business:

Background:

How will your company be set up legally?

Who will own your business?

What is your mission statement?

Where will your business be located?

Who is the target market?

Marketing:

How will you market your services and products to mothers?

How will you market your services and products to the general public?

How will you market your business to businesses/healthcare providers that may be referral sources?

Will you pay for advertising?

What social media will you use?

What other forms of marketing will you engage in?

Finance:

How will you finance your business?

How much will you charge for your services?

How much will you charge for your products?

What accounting method will you use?

How will you make your business profitable?

Congratulations! You've got a business plan. Now, go make it happen!

References

Ahmed, A. H., & Ouzzani, M. (2012). Interactive web-based breastfeeding monitoring: Feasibility, usability, and acceptability. *J Hum Lact, 28*, 468-475.

Ajmere, H. (2014). *Infographic: Social media stats for 2013*. Retrieved from http://www.digitalbuzzblog.com

American Medical Association (AMA). (2010). *AMA policy: Professionalism in the use of social media*. Retrieved from http://www.ama-assn.org/ama/pub/news/news/social-media-policy.page

American Psychological Association (APA). (2014). *Practitioner pointer: Does the use of Skype raise HIPAA compliance issues?* Retrieved from http://www.apapracticecentral.org/update/2014/04-24/skype-hipaa.aspx

Anderson, G. (n.d.). *Inspirational quote of the day archives*. Retrieved from http://www.famous-quotes-and-quotations.com/greg_anderson_author_1.html

Audelo, L. (2014). Connecting with today's mothers. *Clinical Lactation, 5*(1), 16-19. doi: 10.1891/2158-0782.5.1.16

Bailey, L. (1999). Refracted selves? A study of changes in self-identity in the transition to motherhood. *Sociology, 33*(2), 335-352. doi: 10.1177.S0038038599000206

Bank of America. (2013). *Small business owner report 2013*. Retrieved from http://about.bankofamerica.com/assets/pdf/small-business-infographics/Spring_2013_Small_Business_Owner_Report.pdf

Barrett, C. (2011). Healthcare providers may violate HIPAA by using mobile devices to communicate with patients, *ABA Health eSource, 8*(2). Retrieved from http://www.americanbar.org/content/newsletter/publications/aba_health_esource_home/aba_health_law_esource_1110_barrett.html

Beesley, C. (2012). *How to price your small business' products and services*. Retrieved from http://www.sba.gov/blogs/how-price-your-small-business-products-and-services

Bernhardt, J.M., & Felter, E.M. (2004). Online pediatric information seeking among mothers of young children: Results from a qualitative study using focus groups. *J Med Internet Res, 6*(1), e7. doi: 10.2196/jmir.6.1.e7

Bullas, J. (2014). *22 social media facts and statistics you should know in 2014*. Retrieved from http://www.jeffbullas.com/2014/01/17/20-social-media-facts-and-statistics-you-should-know-in-2014/

Business Dictionary. (2014). *Return on investment*. Retrieved from

http://www.businessdictionary.com/definition/return-on-investment-ROI.html

Centers for Disease Control and Prevention (CDC). (2013). *Recommended vaccines for healthcare workers*. Retrieved from http://www.cdc.gov/vaccines/adults/rec-vac/hcw.html

Couch, A. (2014). Creating order from chaos: 9 great ideas for managing your computer files. Retrieved from http://www.makeuseof.com/tag/creating-order-chaos-9-great-ideas-managing-computer-files/

Daly Enterprises Inc. (2014). *Mobile lactation consultant.* Retrieved from http://www.mobilelactationconsultant.com/Lactation-Consultant-Software.aspx

Department of Health and Human Services (DHHS). (2014). *How to apply for an NPI.* Retrieved from https://nppes.cms.hhs.gov/NPPES/Welcome.do

Department of Health and Human Services, Centers for Disease Control and Prevention. (2012). *Audience insights: Communicating to moms.* Retrieved from http://www.cdc.gov/healthcommunication/audience/index.html

Department of Health and Human Services. (2006). *HIPAA security guidance.* Retrieved from http://www.hhs.gov/ocr/privacy/hipaa/administrative/securityrule/remoteuse.pdf

Drentea, P., & Moren-Cross, J.L. (2005). Social capital and social support on the web: The case of an internet mother site. *Sociology of Health & Illness, 27*(7), 920-943. doi: 10.1111/j.1467-95666.2005.00464x

Dunham, P.J., Hurshman, A., Litwin, E., Gresella, J., Ellsworth, C., & Dodd, P.W.D. (1998). Computer-mediated social support: Single young mothers as a model system. *Am J Community Psychology, 26*(2), 281-306. doi: 10.1023/A:1022132720104

Dworkin, G. (1988). *The theory and practice of autonomy.* Cambridge, England: Cambridge University Press.

Edlink. (2014). *Peer learning circles.* Retrieved from http://www.theedlink.org/peer-learning

Entrepreneur Idea Dads. (2011). *How long does it take to become profitable?* Retrieved from http://www.entrepreneurideadads.com/2011/03/how-long-does-it-take-to-become-profitable/

Elsyek, H. (1936). A syndrome produced by nocuos [sic] agents. *Nature, 138,* 32.

Eysenbach, G. (2011). How strong are passwords used to protect personal health information in clinical trials? *J Med Internet Res, 12*(1), e18.

Fleschner, S. (2008). Counseling across generations: Bridging the baby boomer, generations X, and generations Y gap. *VISTAS,* article 14, 139-148. Retrieved from http://www.counselingoutfitters.com/vistas/vistas08/Fleschner_Article_14.pdf

Grant, K.E., Compas, B.E., Stuhimacher, A.F., Thurm, A.E., McMahon, S.D., & Halpert, J. A. (2003). Stressors and child and adolescent psychopathology: Moving from markers to mechanisms of risk. *Psychological Bulletin, 129*(3), 447. doi: 10.1037/0033-2909.129.3.447

Gross, A. (2011). Beware of patient information on smartphones. *HIPAA Secure Now!,* May 25, 2011. [Web blog post]. Retrieved from http://www.hipaasecurenow.com/?s=beware+of+patient+information+on+smartphones

Gunn, E.P. (2011). When to hire a bookkeeper or accountant. Retrieved from http://www.entrepreneur.com/article/219917

Gutowski, J.L. (2012). *Reimbursement: Questions and answers for IBCLCs.* Retrieved from http://
uslca.org/wp-content/uploads/2013/02/Reimbursement_FAQ_Article_for_
USLCA_6-2012_v2.pdf

Hansen, K. (2014). FAQs about job-seeker thank-you letters. *Quinessential Careers.* Retrieved
from http://www.quintcareers.com/thank_you_letters.html

Harden, S. (2014). *Social networking statistics.* Retrieved from http://www.statisticbrain.com/
social-networking-statistics/

Hayden, B. (2013). *Pinterest marketing guide: How to get more traffic and more sales using the
power of pinterest.* Retrieved from http://www.bethhayden.com/wp-content/
uploads/2012/07/PInterestMarketingGuide.pdf

Hjemdahl, P. (2002). Stress and the metabolic syndrome: An interesting but enigmatic
association. *Circulation, 106*(21), 2634. doi: 10.1161/01.CIR.0000041502.43564.79

Hyatt, M. (2007). *Email etiquette 101.* Retrieved from
http://www.michaelhyatt.com/e-mail-etiquette-101.html

IHS Inc. (2014). *A dedicated study on telehealth that provides detailed analysis of the world market.*
Retrieved from http://assets.fiercemarkets.com/public/newsletter/fiercehealthit/
abstract-ihshome-health-technology-2014.pdf

Internal Revenue Service (IRS). (2014). *Schedule C, Profit or Loss from Business, Form 1040.*
Retrieved from http://www.irs.gov/uac/Schedule-C-(Form-1040),-Profit-or-Loss-
From-Business

Internal Revenue Service (IRS). (2013). *Publication 587: Business use of your home.* Retrieved
from http://www.irs.gov/publications/p587/ar02.html

International Lactation Consultant Association (ILCA). (2013). *The standards of practice for
International Board Certified Lactation Consultants.* Retrieved from http://www.ilca.org/
files/resources/ilca_publications/Standard_of_Practice.pdf

Johnson, C. (1992). Coping with compassion fatigue. *Nursing, 22*(4), 118-120.

Jolly, L., & Ryan, M. (2014). *Resources for lactation professions - Lactation consultant documentation
forms.* Retrieved from http://www.bayareabreastfeeding.net/Blank.html

Kabat-Zinn, J. (2014). *Welcome to mindful living programs.* Retrieved from http://www.
mindfullivingprograms.com/index.php

Kaplan, R. (2012). *How IBCLCs can make an impact through social media.* Retrieved from http://
lactationmatters.org/?s=How+IBCLCs+can+make+an+impact+through+social+m
edia

Kennis, L. (2012). *25 things that make you look dumb on LinkedIn.* Retrieved from http://
www.business2community.com/linkedin/25-things-that-make-you-look-dumb-on-
linkedin-0559620

Lang Kosa, J. (2013). *Taking my private practice "paperless."* Retrieved from http://www.lactationmatters.org/2013/taking-my-private-practice-paperless/

Lindsey, P. (2014). *ICD-10 Lactation Visit Receipt, a professional receipt of lactation services: a "lactation superbill."* Retrieved from http://www.patlc.com/LVR

Macnab, I., Rojjanasrirat, W., & Sanders, S. (2012). *Breastfeeding and telehealth. Jour Hum Lact, 28*(4), 446-449. doi: 10.1177/0890334412460512

McCall, K. (2000). *Home-based business: Is it for you?* Retrieved from http://www.inc.com/articles/2000/03/17919.html

McCann, A.D., & McCulloch, J. (2012). Establishing an online and social media presence for your IBCLC practice. *J Hum Lact, 28*, 450-454. doi: 10.1177/0890334412461304

McEwen, B.S. (1998). Protective and damaging effects of stress mediators. *New England Journal of Medicine, 338*(3), 171. doi: 10.1056/NEJM199801153380307

Morningstar.com. (2014). *Industry returns.* Retrieved from http://news.morningstar.com/stockReturns/CapWtdIndustryReturns.html

Myler, E., West, D., & Lisimachio, J. (2014). *Lactation charting forms.* Retrieved from http://www.mahalamom.com

Narkiewicz, K. (2002). Obesity-related hypertension: Relevance of vascular responses to mental stress. [Editorial comment]. *Journal of Hypertension, 20*(7), 1277.

Oblinger, D. (2003). Boomers and gen-Xers & millennials: Understanding the new students. *EDUCAUSEreview*, July/Aug, 37-48.

O'Connor, H., & Madge, E. (2004). 'My mum's thirty years out of date': The role of the internet in the transition to motherhood. *Community, Work & Family, 7*(3), 351-369. doi: 10.1080/1366880042000295754

O'Hare, E., Shaw, D.L., Tierney, K.J., Kim, E.M., Levine, A.S., & Shepard, R.A. (2004). Behavioral and neurochemical mechanisms of the action of mild stress in the enhancement of feeding. *Behavioral Neuroscience, 118*(1), 173. doi: 10.1037/0735-7044.118.1.173

Online Etymology Dictionary. (n.d.). *Compassion.* Retrieved from http://dictionary.reference.com/browse/compassion

Parkes, K. (2004). *Psychophysiological effects of stress.* Unpublished work.

Pate, B. (2009). A systematic review of the effectiveness of breastfeeding intervention delivery methods. *JOGNN, 38*(6), 642-653. doi: 10.1111/j.1552-6909.2009.01068.x

Plantin, L., & Daneback, K. (2009). Parenthood, information and support on the internet: A literature review of research on parents and professionals online. *BMC Family Practice, 10*, 34-46. doi: 10.1186/1471-2296-10-34

Porterfield, A., Khare, P. & Vahl, A. (2011). *Facebook marketing all-in-one for dummies.* Hobeken, NJ: Wiley Publishing Inc.

Rojjanasrirat, W., Nelson, E., & Wamback, K. A. (2012). A pilot study of home-based videoconferencing for breastfeeding support. *J Hum Lact;* 28: 464-467.

Ross, M.S. (2012). *#Pinterest makes top 50 website list.* Retrieved from h t t p : / / w w w . searchenginejournal.com/pinterest-makes-top-50-website-list/50592/

SANS Institute. (2003). *A consumer guide for personal file and disk encryption programs.* Retrieved from http://www.sans.org/reading-room/whitepapers/vpns/consumer-guide-personal-file-disk-encryption-programs-884

Santana, G. (2014). *Top 10 ways to be successful in both business and life. Business Know-How.* Retrieved from http://www.businessknowhow.com/growth/bizlife.htm

Schwartz, A.R., Gerin, W., Davidson, K.W., Pickering, T.G., Brosschot, J.F., Thayer, J F.,

et al. (2003). Toward a causal model of cardiovascular responses to stress and the

development of cardiovascular disease. *Psychosomatic Medicine, 65*(1), 22.

Shaikh, U., & Scott, B.J. (2005). Extent, accuracy, and credibility of breastfeeding information on the internet. *J Hum Lact, 21,* 175-183. doi:10.1177/0890334405275824

Snoke, C. (2014). *Data backup software review.* Retrieved from http://data-backup-software-review.toptenreviews.com

Spector, N., & Kappel, D.M. (2012). Guidelines for using electronic and social media: The regulatory perspective. *OJIN: Online J of Issues in Nurs, 17*(3), manuscript 1. Retrieved from http://www.nursingworld.org/MainMenuCategories/ANAMarketplace/ANAPeriodicals/OJIN/TableofContents/Vol-17-2012/No3-Sept-2012/Guidelines-for-Electronic-and-Social-Media.html doi:10.3912/OJIN.Vol17Nov03Man01

Strauss, W. (2005, Sept 10-14). Talking about their generations. *The School Administrator.*

Steckler, T. (2001). The molecular neurobiology of stress-evidence from genetic and epigenetic models. *Behavioral Pharmacology, 12*(6-7), 381.

Stevens, P.S. (2014). *Small business accounting software review 2014.* Retrieved from http://accounting-software-review.toptenreviews.com

Thurman, S.E., & Allen, P.J. (2008). Integrating lactation consultants into primary health care services: Are lactation consultants affecting breastfeeding success? *Pediatr Nurs, 34*(5), 419-425.

Topping, K.J. (2005). Trends in peer learning. *Education Psychology, 25*(6), 631-645.

Tunajek, S. (2007). Peer support: Validity and benefit. *AANA NewsBulletin, 5,* 29-31.

USDA. (2014). *WIC program: FY 2013.* Retrieved from

http://www.fns.usda.gov/pd/wic- program

Versel, N. (2012, June 15). Off-the-shelf smartphones meet few HIPAA, MU security requirements. *Mobihealthnews.* Retrieved from http://mobihealthnews.com/17663/off-the-shelf-smartphones-meet-few-hipaa-mu-security-requirements/

Wasserman, E. 2009). *How to price business services.* Retrieved from http://www.inc.com/guides/price-your-services.html

Wilson, J.L. (2010). *The best small business accounting software.* Retrieved from http://www.pcmag.com/article2/0,2817,2363725,00.asp

Wolynn, T. (2012). Using social media to promote and support breastfeeding. *Breastfeeding Medicine, 7*(5), 364-366. doi: 10.1089.bfm.2012.0085

World Health Organization (WHO). (1981). *International code of marketing of breast-milk substitutes.* Retrieved from http://www.who.int/nutrition/publications/infantfeeding/9241541601/en/

World Health Organization (WHO). (2011). *Status report on country implementation of the International Code of Marketing of Breast-milk Substitutes.* Retrieved from http://apps.who.int/iris/bitstream/10665/85621/1/9789241505987_eng.pdf

Zweig, J., Stepanchuk, I., Swyter, H., Smith, C., & DiLauro, M. (2013, October 24). *5 accounting mistakes that put your small business at risk.* Retrieved from http://www.freshbooks.com/blog/2013/10/24/5-accounting-mistakes/

Appendix A
National and International
Breastfeeding Organizations

Organization	Website
Australian Breastfeeding Association	www.breastfeeding.asn.au/
Baby-Friendly Hospital Initiative Australia	www.babyfriendly.org.au
Baby-Friendly Hospital Initiative Canada	www.breastfeedingcanada.ca/
Baby-Friendly Hospital Initiative Ireland	www.babyfriendly.ie
Baby-Friendly Hospital Initiative Ireland	www.ihph.ie/babyfriendlyinitiative/
Baby-Friendly Hospital Initiative Lautoka, Fiji	www.pacifichealthdialog.org.fi
Baby-Friendly Hospital Initiative Netherlands	www.zvb.borstvoeding.nl
Baby-Friendly Hospital Initiative New Zealand	www.babyfriendly.org.nz/
Baby-Friendly Hospital Initiative Switzerland	www.allaiter.ch
Baby-Friendly Hospital Initiative United Arab Emigrants	www.dha.gov.ae/EN/Facilities/Hospitals/ AlWaslHospital/PatientsGuide/HealthEducation/ BabyFriendlyHospitalInitiative/Pages/default.aspx
Baby-Friendly USA	www.babyfriendlyusa.org/
Canadian Lactation Consultant Association	www.ilca.org/i4a/pages/index.cfm?pageid=3519
ILCA Affiliate-Germany	www.bdl-stillen.de/
ILCA Affiliate-Great Britain	www.lcgb.org/
ILCA Affiliate-Israel	www.iaclc.org.il/
ILCA Affiliate-Italy	www.aicpam.org/
ILCA Affiliate-Japan	www.jalc-net.jp/
International Board of Lactation Consultant Examiners	www.iblce.org

International Lactation Consultant Association	www.ilca.org
La Leche League International	www.llli.org/
Lactation Consultants of Australia and New Zealand	www.lcanz.org
Lactitude France	www.lactitude.com/text/Ress_Web-FR.html
Natural Feeding Consultants of Russia	www.akev.ru/
UNICEF Baby-Friendly Hospital Initiative Hong Kong	www.babyfriendly.org.hk/en/
UNICEF Baby-Friendly Hospital Initiative UK	www.unicef.org.uk/babyfriendly
United States Breastfeeding Committee	www.usbreastfeeding.org
United States Lactation Consultant Association	www.uslca.org
World Alliance for Breastfeeding Action	www.waba.org.my/
World Health Organization–Baby-Friendly Hospital Initiative	www.who.int/nutrition/topics/bfhi/en/

Appendix B
U.S. State Breastfeeding Coalitions

State	Website
Alabama	www.alabamabreastfeeding.org
Alaska	www.alaskabreastfeeding.com
Arizona	www.azbreastfeeding.org
Arkansas	www.arbfc.org
California	www.californiabreastfeeding.org
Colorado	www.cobfc.org
Connecticut	www.breastfeedingct.org
Delaware	www.delawarebreastfeeding.org
District of Columbia	www.dcbfc.org
Florida	www.flbreastfeeding.org
Georgia	www.georgiabreastfeedingcoalition.org
Hawaii	www.breastfeedinghawaii.org
Idaho	www.facebook.com/ISBC.network
Illinois	www.illinoisbreastfeeding.org
Iowa	www.iabreastfeeding.org
Kansas	www.ksbreastfeeding.org
Kentucky	www.breastfeedingkentucky.com
Louisiana	www.louisianabreastfeedingcoalition.org
Maine	www.mainestatebreastfeedingcoalition.org
Maryland	www.marylandbreastfeedingcoalition.org
Massachusetts	www.massbreastfeeding.org
Michigan	www.mibfnetwork.org
Minnesota	www.mnbreastfeedingcoalition.org
Mississippi	www.msbfc.org
Missouri	www.mobreastfeeding.org
Montana	www.mtbreastfeedingcoalition.weebly.com
Nebraska	www.nebreastfeeding.org
Nevada	www.nevadabreastfeeding.org
New Hampshire	www.nhbreastfeedingtaskforce.org
New Jersey	www.breastfeedingnj.org
New Mexico	www.breastfeedingnewmexico.org
New York	www.nysbreastfeeding.org
North Carolina	www.ncbfc.org

North Dakota	www.ndhealth.gov/breastfeeding/?id=66
Ohio	www.ohiobreastfeedingalliance.org
Oklahoma	www.okbreastfeeding.org
Oregon	www.breastfeedingor.org
Pennsylvania	www.pabreastfeeding.org
Rhode Island	www.ribreastfeeding.org
South Carolina	www.scbreastfeedingcoalition.org
South Dakota	www.sdbreastfeedingcoalition.com
Tennessee	www.breastfeeding.tn.gov/
Texas	www.texasbreastfeedingcoalition.org/
Utah	www.utahbreastfeeding.org
Vermont	www.tcass@vah.vt.us
Washington	www.withinreachwa.org/
West Virginia	www.wvbfa.com
Wisconsin	www.wibreastfeeding.com
Wyoming	www.wyobreastfeedingcoalition.org

Appendix C
Professional Organizations and Sources

Organization	Website
Academy for Breastfeeding Medicine	www.bfmed.org
Academy of Lactation Policy and Practice	www.talpp.org/
Academy of Nutrition and Dietetics	www.eatright.org/About/Content.aspx?id=8377
Adoptive Breastfeeding Resources	www.fourfriends.com
American Academy of Family Practice	www.aafp.org/about/policies/all/breastfeeding.html
American Academy of Ob/Gyns	www.acog.org
American Academy of Pediatricians	www.aap.org
American College of Nurse Midwives	www.midwife.org/
American Congress of Obstetricians and Gynecologists	www.acog.org
American Public Health Association	www.apha.org/
Association for Pre- & Perinatal Psychology	www.birthpsychology.com/apppah/index.html
Association of Women's Health, Obstetric, and Neonatal Nurses	www.awhonn.org
Australian National Breastfeeding Strategy	www.health.gov.au/pubhlth/strateg/brfeed/
Baby Milk Action-IBFAN UK	www.babymilkaction.org/
Best Start	www.beststart.org/resources/breastfeeding/index.html
Biological Nurturing	www.biologicalnurturing.com/
Breastfeeding and Human Lactation Study Center	http://www.urmc.rochester.edu/childrens-hospital/neonatology/lactation.aspx
Breastfeeding Promotion Network of India	www.bpni.org/

Breastmilk Solutions, Dr. Jane Morton	www.breastmilksolutions.com/
Center for Breastfeeding Information (CBI)	www.llli.org/cbi/cbi.html
Centers for Disease Control and Prevention	www.cdc.gov/breastfeeding/
Coalition for Improving Maternity Services	www.motherfriendly.org/
European Milk Bank Association (EMBA)	www.europeanmilkbanking.com
Hale Publishing	www.ibreastfeeding.com/
Healthy Mothers/Healthy Babies	www.hmhb.org
Healthy People 2020	www.healthypeople.gov/2020/default.aspx
HHS Blueprint for Action on Breastfeeding (U.S. Department of Health and Human Services)	http://womenshealth.gov/archive/breastfeeding/ programs/blueprints/bluprntbk2.pdf
Human Milk Banking Association of North America	www.hmbana.org/
INFACT Canada	www.infactcanada.ca/
Infant and Young Child Feeding in Emergency Situation	www.wellstart.org/Infant_feeding_emergency.pdf
InfantRisk Center (Dr. Tom Hale)	www.infantrisk.com/
International Baby-Food Action Network	www.ibfan.org/
International Society for Research in Human Milk and Lactation	http://isrhml.net/
Jack Newman, MD, IBCLC	www.drjacknewman.com
Low Milk Supply	www.lowmilksupply.org
Linkages	www.linkagesproject.org/
March of Dimes	www.marchofdimes.com/
Medications and Mothers' Milk	www.neonatal.ttuhsc.edu/lact/
MICROMEDEX Healthcare Series	http://www.micromedex.com/products/hcs/
National Alliance for Breastfeeding Advocacy	www.nababreastfeeding.com
National Healthy Mothers/ Healthy Babies Coalition	www.hmhb.org/
Nice Breastfeeding (Dr. Frank Nice)	www.nicebreastfeeding.com/
Nursing Mothers Council	www.nursingmothers.org/

Pollywog-Infant Reflux, Colic, and Baby Gas	www.pollywogbaby.com
Stanford University Breastfeeding	www.newborns.stanford.edu/breastfeeding
Surgeon General Call to Action to Support Breastfeeding	www.surgeongeneral.gov/topics/breastfeeding/index.html
UNICEF	www.unicef.org/nutrition/index_breastfeeding.html
U.S. National Library of Medicine	www.nlm.nih.gov/
Wellstart, International	www.wellstart.org
WIC Program	www.fns.usda.gov/wic/women-infants-and-children-wic
William Sears, M.D.	www.askdrsears.com
World Health Organization	www.who.int/en/

Appendix D
Research Sites

Site	Website
BioMed Central	www.biomedcentral.com
Centre for Reviews and Dissemination	www.crd.your.ac.uk
Directory of Open Access Journals	www.doaj.org
Google Scholar	http://scholar.google.com/
InfantRisk Center	www.infantrisk.com/
International Breastfeeding Journal	www.internationalbreastfeedingjournal.com
Journal of the American Medical Association	www.subs.ama-assn.org
Lactmed	www.nlm.nih.gov/news/lactmed_announce_06.html
Lactnet	www.lsoft.com/scripts/wl.exe?SL1 =LACTNET&H=COMMUNITY. LSOFT.COM
Medline-National Library of Medicine	www.ncbi.nlm.nih.gov/entrez/ query.fcgi
Meds and More Newsletter	www.ibreastfeeding.com
On-line Journal of Nursing Informatics	www.hhdev.psu.edu/nurs/ojni/dm/
PubGet	www.pubget.com
PubMed	www.ncbi.nih.gov/pubmed/
TOXNET - Toxicology Data Network	http://www.toxnet.nlm.nih.gov/ cgi-n/sis/htmlgen?LACT

Appendix E
Email Lists & Blogs

Email List/Blog	Website
Amie Urban blog	http://www.phdinparenting.com/
Attachment Parenting blog	http://attachmentparenting.org/blog/
Babyconferences	http://www.breastfeedingconferences.com.au/
Best For Babes	http://www.bestforbabes.org/the-latest-on-latching
Best For Babes: 6 different blogs	http://www.bestforbabes.org/blog/
Biological Nurturing	http://www.biologicalnurturing.com/
Blacktating blog	http://blacktating.blogspot.com/
Blog: "15 Tricks of Formula Companies"	http://www.thealphaparent.com/2011/10/15-tricks-of-formula-companies.html
Blog: Academy of Breastfeeding Medicine	http://bfmed.wordpress.com/
Blog: "Diary of a Lactation Failure"	http://diaryofalactationfailure.blogspot.com/
Diane Cassar-Uhl blog	http://dianaibclc.com/
Dispelling Breastfeeding Myths blog	http://thelactivist.blogspot.com/
Dr. Miriam Labbock	http://enabling-breastfeeding.blogspot.com/
Dr. Jane Morton	http://newborns.stanford.edu/Breastfeeding/ABCs.html#GettingStarted
IBCLC-PP	https://groups.yahoo.com/neo/groups/IBCLC-PP/
Katie Hindi blog	http://mammalssuck.blogspot.com/
Lactation Matters:	http://lactationmatters.wordpress.com/
Lactconnect Breastfeeding blog	http://lactconnect.blogspot.com/
Lactnet	http://community.lsoft.com/scripts/WA-LSOFTDONATIONS.exe?A0=LACTNET
Lactivist blog	http://thelactivist.blogspot.com/
Lactivist Leanings blog	http://www.lactivistleanings.com/
LactPsych	https://groups.yahoo.com/neo/groups/LactPsych/

Leigh Anne O'Connor blog	http://mamamilkandme.com/
Milkyway blog	http://milkywaymilkshare.blog.com/
Nancy Mohrbacher Breastfeeding Reporter	http://www.nancymohrbacher.com/
Postpartum Progress blog	http://www.postpartumprogress.com/
Robin Kaplan blog	http://sdbfc.com/blog/
The Beautiful Letdown blog	http://beautifulletdown.net/
The Leaky Boob blog	http://theleakyboob.com/

Appendix F
Breast Pumps and Accessories

Company	Products
Ameda Ameda, Inc. 485 Half Day Road, Suite 320 Buffalo Grove, IL 60089 Phone: 877-992-6332 / 877-99-AM-EDA www.ameda.com orders@ameda.com **Ameda International Office** Mechelsesteenweg 251 B-1800 Vilvoorde Belgium Phone: +32-2-304-52-79 internationalsales@ameda.com **AMEDA (Shanghai) Trading Co., Ltd.** B3001-02 City Center, 100 Zunyi Road, Changning District, Shanghai, China, 200051 Phone: 400-030-0525 www.ameda.com.cn	Ameda Platinum® Breast Pump Ameda Elite™ Breast Pump Ameda Purely Yours® Double Electric Breast Pump Ameda Lactaline™ Double Electric Breast Pump Ameda One-Hand Manual Pump Ameda CustomFit Flange System™ Ameda NoShow Premium™ Nursing Pads and reusable nursing pads Ameda Comfort Gel™ Extended Use Hydrogel Pads Ameda ComfortLan™ 100% Pure Lanolin. Nipple Shields DuoShell™ Breast Shells and accessory parts

Bailey Medical 2216 Sunset Dr. Los Osos, CA 93402 Phone: 805-528-5781/800-413-3216 Fax: 805-528-1461 www.baileymed.com folks@baileymed.com	Deluxe Nurture III Breast Pump Basic Nurture III Breast Pump Super Shields- Medium B/C Cup (23-29mm; pair) Super Shields–Extra Large D+ Cup (35+mm; pair) Milk Storage Bags 100% Cotton Breast Pads (4) M. & B.-A (Milk And Baby)–Herbal Blend–1 oz & 4 oz Air-Dry Accessory Bag
Hygeia Hygeia Medical Group II 1375 S. Acacia Avenue Fullerton, CA 92831 Phone: 714-515-7571 or 888-786-7466 Fax: 714-494-8571 www.hygeiainc.com customer.service@hygeiababy.com	Enjoye™ Breast Pump with Internal Battery Enjoye™ LBI Breast Pump with Deluxe Tote Set Enjoye™ Breast Pump without Internal Battery EnDeare™ Breast Pump Hygeia Two-Hand Manual Breast Pump EnHande™ One-Hand Manual Breast Pump Washable Nursing Pads Hygeia Hand Expression Cup Set Breast Milk Storage Bags Transitional Supplementation Feeder

Lansinoh	Signature Pro™ Double Electric Breast Pump
Lansinoh Laboratories, Inc.	Affinity Pro™ Double Electric Breast Pump
333 North Fairfax Street, Suite 400	Affinity® Double Electric Breast Pump
Alexandria, VA, 22314	Manual Breast Pump
Phone: 877-366-1182	Comfort Express™ Manual Breast Pump
www.lansinoh.com	Large Comfort Fit Flanges
	Simple Wishes™ Hands-Free Pumping Bra
	Breastmilk Storage Bags
	HPA® Lanolin
	Disposable Nursing Pads
	Ultra-Soft Disposable Nursing Pads
	LatchAssist® Nipple Everter
	Soothies® by Lansinoh® Gel Pads
	THERA°PEARL® 3-in-1 Breast Therapy
Mamivac	Mamivac® Sensitive-C Hospital Grade Pump
KaWeCo GmbH	Mamivac® Sensitive-Cfh Hospital Grade Pump
Gerlinger Straße 36-38	Mamivac® Lactive
71254 Ditzingen, Germany	Mamivac® Easy Manual Pump
Phone: +49 (0) 71 56 - 1 76 02 -100	Mamivac® Nursing Pads
Fax: +49 (0) 71 56 - 1 76 02 - 500	Mamivac® Thermo-Pack
www.kaweco.de	Mamilan® Breast Cream
info@kaweco.de	Conical nipple shields
	S–Small; D=18 mm
	M–Medium; D=20 mm
	L–Large; D=28 mm
	Cherry-shaped nipple shields
	S–Small; D=18 mm
	M–Medium; D=22 mm

Medela	Symphony® Breastpump
Medela, Inc. Breastfeeding US	Symphony® Preemie+™ Breastpump
1101 Corporate Drive	Lactina® Select Breastpump
McHenry, IL 60050	Freestyle® Breastpump
Phone: 800-435-8316	Pump In Style® Advanced
Fax: 800-995-7867	Swing™ Breastpump
www.medelabreastfeedingus.com	Pump In Style Advanced Breastpump Starter Set (insurance pump)
	PersonalFit™ Breastshields
	Quick Clean™ Breastmilk Removal Soap
	Quick Clean™ Breastpump & Accessory Wipes
	Quick Clean™ Micro-Steam Bags
	Easy Expression™ Bustier
	Bras
	BabyWeigh™ II Scale
	Pump & Save Bags
	Supplemental Nursing System™ (SNS™)
	Starter Supplemental Nursing System™ (SNS™) (sterile)
	SpecialNeeds® Feeder
	Mini-SpecialNeeds® Feeder (Sterile)
	SoftFeeder™
	Tender Care™ Lanolin
	Tender Care™ Hydrogel Pads
	Disposable Nursing Pads
	Washable Bra Pads
	Contact Nipple Shields
	SoftShells™
	TheraShells™

Philips Avent P.O. Box 77900 1070 MX Amsterdam The Netherlands Phone: 800-542-8368 www.usa.philips.com/c-m-mo/ philips-avent-and-your-baby	AVENT Comfort Double Electric Breast Pump AVENT Comfort Single Electric Breast Pump AVENT Comfort manual breast pump AVENT Large Massage Cushion Accessory AVENT Breastcare Thermo pads AVENT Niplette AVENT Disposable Breast Pads AVENT Nipple Protectors AVENT Comfort Breast Shell Set AVENT Breast Milk Storage Bags
Simplisse (now Dr. Brown's) Handi-Craft Company 4433 Fyler Ave. St. Louis, Missouri 63116 Phone: 800-778-9001 Fax: 314-773-9273 www.drbrownsbaby.com	Double Electric Breast Pump Manual Breast Pump Breastmilk Storage Bags Breastmilk Storage Tray Disposable Breast Pads Washable Breast Pads Gia* Breastfeeding Pillows Lanolin-Free Nipple Cream HydroGel Soothing Pads

Appendix G
Other Supplies

Company	Products
A to Z Vet Supply 9876 Hwy. 22 Dresden, TN 38225 Phone: 800-979-2869 Fax: 800-979-2870 www.atozvetsupply.com	Variety of feeding tubes Monoject syringes Monoject Curved Tip syringes
California Veterinary Supply 891 W. Indole St. Pahrump, NV 89048 Phone: 800-366-3047 Fax: 775-727-4498 www.calvetsupply.com help@calvetsupply.com	Variety of feeding tubes Variety of syringes Curved tip syringes
Medline Industries One Medline Place Mundelein, Illinois 60060 Phone: 847-949-5500 Fax: 800-351-1512 www.medline.com service@medline.com	Variety of feeding tubes Variety of syringes Curved tip syringes
Lact-Aid International, Inc. P.O. Box 1066 Athens, TN 37371-1066 Phone (USA): 866-866-1239 Phone (outside USA): 423-744-9090 Fax: 423-744-9090 www.lact-aid.com	Lact-Aid Nursing Trainer System

Appendix H
Herbal Galactogogue Sources

Company	Product
Motherlove Herbal Company 1420 Riverside Ave, Suite 114 Fort Collins, CO 80524 Phone: 970-493-2892 Fax: 970-224-4844 www.motherlove.com mother@motherlove.com	Variety of herbal products for breast-feeding mothers
Oasis Tea Company 1894 East William Street, Suite 4 Carson City, NV 89701 www.Oasisteacompany.com info@oasisteacompany.com	Oasis Prolactation Tea and Power Booster
Phoenix Herb Company 4305 Main St Kansas City, MO 64111 Phone: 816-531-8327 www.phoenixherb.com	Herbs, spices, and teas
Stony Mountain Botanicals P.O. Box 106 Loudonville, OH 44842 Phone: 419-938-6353 www.wildroots.com	Essential oils, herbs, spices
Traditional Medicinals 4515 Ross Road Sebastopol, CA 95472 Phone: 800-543-4372 www.traditionalmedicinals.com traditionalmedicinals@worldpantry.com	Variety of teas

Appendix I
Nursing Pillows, Slings, Scales, and Other Products

Company	Product
Balboa Baby & Co. LLC 3001 Red Hill Avenue, Suite 5-103 Costa Mesa, CA 92626 Phone: 949-200-7541/866-465-7075 Fax: 866-910-1710 www.balboababy.com info@balboababy.com	Slings, nursing covers, nursing pillows, high chair covers, stroller liners
The Boppy Company 560 Golden Ridge Road, Ste. 150 Golden, CO 80401 Phone: 888-772-6779 www.boppy.com cbeinfo@boppy.com	Feeding pillows, baby chair, newborn lounger, slipcovers
Diva-Milano LilyRose Style (UK) LLP 277 Gray's Inn Road London WC1X8QF United Kingdom www.diva-milano.com info@diva-milano.com	Slings, nursing tops
DOUBLE BLESSINGS 2739 Via Orange Way, Suite #117 Spring Valley, CA 91978 USA Phone: 800-584-8946 Fax: 619-741-8624 www.doubleblessings.com	Nursing pillow for multiples, bibs, slings

EARTH MAMA ANGEL BABY 9866 SE Empire Court Clackamas, OR 97015 Phone: 503-607-0607 Fax: 503-607-0667 www.earthmamaangelbaby.com/	Natural, non-toxin nipple butter, baby balm, soaps, herbs
HOTSLINGS Mother's Lounge LLC Phone: 801-768-9440 Fax: 801-753-7366 www.hotslings.com/	Slings
KIINDE Kiinde LLC P.O. Box 8804 Warwick, RI 02888 Phone: 401-223-2977 www.kiinde.com/ sales@kiinde.com	Breastmilk storage system
Leachco PO Box 717 Ada, Oklahoma 74821 Phone: 800-525-1050/580-436-1142 www.leachco.com	Nursing pillows, covers, bibs, bathers, safety items
LILYPADZ Phone: 800-640-LILY www.lilypadz.com/	Silicone nursing pads
Mother's Lounge 363 W Industrial Dr. Pleasant Grove Utah, 84062 Phone: 800-766-2290 www.motherslounge.com service@motherslounge.com	Wholesale mother & baby product distribution
Sakura Bloom www.sakurabloom.com	Ring slings

SCALESONLINE 4758 Ridge Road #251 Cleveland, Ohio 44144 Phone: 866-856-6100 Fax: 866-458-3068 www.scalesonline.com	Doran Digital Baby Scale, accurate to within 5 grams Healthometer Digital Baby Scale, accurate to within 15 grams Seca Digital Baby Scale, accurate to within 6 grams
Sensible Lines, LLC P.O. Box 813 Lithia, FL 33547 www.Sensiblelines.com info@sensiblelines.com	Milk trays
SWEETPEA RING SLINGS www.sweetpearingsling.com/	Ring slings
TWIN Z Pillow Phone: 603-732-2345 www.twinznursingpillow.com info@twinznursingpillow.com	Nursing pillows for twins
ZANYTOES Custom Slings www.zanytoes.net/	Ring slings
Zenoff Products, Inc. 25 Tamalpias Ave, Suite C San Anselmo, CA 94960 Phone: 415-785-3890 Fax: 415-785-8139 www.mybrestfriend.com info@zenoffprod.com	My Brest Friend nursing and body pillows
Zolowear Slings and Carriers Baby Holdings, Inc. 8525 Jackrabbit Rd, Suite B Houston, TX 77095 Phone: 888-285-0044/832-239-5110 www.zolowear.com	Slings, pouches, and carriers

Index

About the Author

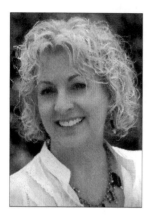

Kathy Parkes has been assisting breastfeeding mothers for over 30 years, first as a volunteer and now as a professional. She lives in San Antonio, Texas with her husband of almost 40 years, Bruce. Her daughter Sarah lives in Houston, TX with her husband and three children. Daughter Jill lives in Austin, TX.

Perspectives in Lactation: Is Private Practice for Me? is Kathy's first book. There will be more topics to come in the Perspectives in Lactation series; watch the www.breastfeedingperspectives.com website for future announcements.

Dear Reader,

Thank you for purchasing and reading this book. I hope you enjoyed it. If so, you can help me reach other readers by writing a review of the book on Amazon.com, ibreastfeeding.com, and/or on my website–www. breastfeedingperspectives.com

Sincerely,

Kathy Parkes

Made in the USA
San Bernardino, CA
31 October 2017